Reviews of The Australian Tea Tree Oil Guide, Third Edition:

"Tea tree oil remedies abound these days – indeed this new 'wonder herb' from the land down under is all the rage this year. You may be surprised to learn that it's actually been around for quite awhile, first mentioned in European journals by Captain Cook in the late 19th century. Author Cynthia Olsen details every facet and application for Melaleuca alternifolia in her book *Australian Tea Tree Oil Guide: First Aid Kit in a Bottle*. A source list and a guide for treating pets with tea tree oil round out the text."

The Herb Quarterly, Winter 1997

"Melaleuca alternifolia, otherwise known as tea tree oil, has become a popular and common ingredient in many cosmetic and personal hygiene products. . . Tea tree oil is a natural antiseptic and fungicide, a dozen times stronger than carbolic acid but far less irritating to the skin. This makes it useful for all kinds of irritation, from dandruff to gingivitis, from bee stings to rashes to acne. This third edition of the guide tells the history of tea tree oil and how it's produced, and doubles as a practitioner's guide in how and when to use it. Also included are a glossary, a bibliography, and a list of resources and suppliers."

NAPRA Review, Holiday 1997

"In contemporary times we suffer from diseases which are puzzling. As modern medicines become less effective against viral and chronic illness and immune deficiencies, we turn to ancient healing modalities. Tea Tree Oil is classified as one of those herbal plant essences that has been known for centuries, but 'forgotten' in our post-war years of so-called miracle drugs.

"Olsen gives us a complete history and guide – with tables to accompany the text – on how, when and where to use this all-purpose and potent oil. She backs up her findings with good sources and personal testimonies, and includes a practitioner's guide to the use of tea tree oil. Definitely a b̶o̶o̶k̶ ̶t̶o̶ ̶k̶e̶e̶p̶ ̶p̶r̶o̶p̶p̶e̶d̶ ̶u̶p̶ ̶i̶n̶ ̶y̶o̶u̶r̶ medicine cabinet or in your treatment r̶o̶o̶m̶

̶s̶, January 1998

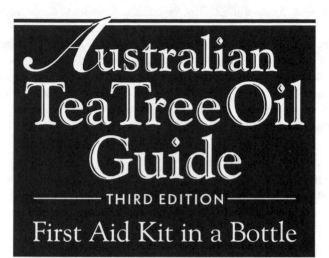

Australian Tea Tree Oil Guide

—— THIRD EDITION ——

First Aid Kit in a Bottle

WITH PHOTOGRAPHS & UPDATED RESOURCE GUIDE

CYNTHIA OLSEN

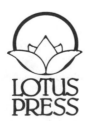

LOTUS PRESS

Herbal medicine has been around for centuries. Ancient cultures have drawn from nature the means to implement these herbal remedies to use as medicine for healing.

Although tea tree oil has been studied for most of this century, it is still important to use common sense when experimenting with herbs or essential oils such as tea tree. If adverse reactions occur, discontinue use. *The author does not imply any cure or medical solutions when using the information in this book. It is always advisable to consult with a qualified professional health practitioner before engaging in any self treatment.*

Cover design and execution: Paul Bond, Art & Soul Design
Editing, page composition and book design: Susan Tinkle
Illustrations: Susan Tinkle
Photos courtesy of: Australian Plantations
Cover photo: Main Camp Tea Tree Oil Group

Published by:

Lotus Press
PO Box 325
Twin Lakes, WI 53181
email: lotuspress@lotuspress.com
website: www.lotuspress.com

Printed in the United States of America
10 9 8 7 6 5 4 3 2

Library of Congress Cataloging in Publication Data
Olsen, Cynthia B.
    Australian tea tree oil guide : first aid kit in a bottle : with photographs and updated resource guide / Cynthia Olsen. — Rev. 3rd ed.
        p. cm.
    Includes bibliographical references and index.
    ISBN 1-890941-01-8 (pbk.)
    1. Melaleuca alternifolia oil—Therapeutic use.   I. Title.
RM666.M357047 1997b
615'.32376—dc21   98-35973
                                                                                      CIP

Acknowledgements

*T*he third edition of the Guide was made possible because many people contributed, with dedication and professional integrity, to making it a reality. Others have helped produce this updated version, and I would like to acknowledge them here.

Susan Tinkle for editing, organization, and creative skills. Thank you again, my friend. Always a great pleasure to collaborate with you.

Paul Bond of Art & Soul Design, who created such a beautiful cover. I look forward to our next project.

Cheyanne West, for your valuable contribution to the animal care chapter. Thank you for sharing your expertise in the field of natural care for small and large animals.

Erin Wood, my special assistant during the release of the third edition, and Christen Aaron, presently my right-hand person, who is so adept at managing the many details of a small publishing office.

Mark Blumenthal, a true pioneer in the herbal and natural health movement. Thank you for taking time out of your busy life to share your expert advice about herbs and tea tree oil.

Robert Cook, who introduced me to tea tree oil. Through our work in the early years, importing and introducing the oil in this country, I was led to become an author and publisher. Thank you for sharing your vision. Gregory Smith, the detail man, who fine-tuned the 1997 manuscript just before press time. Thank you my friend.

William Branson of Australian Holdings for answering many of my questions regarding the tea tree industry in Australia.

Australian Plantations, for their contribution of the beautiful photographs for the revised edition and updated material on tea tree oil standards.

Main Camp Tea Tree Plantation in Australia, for the valuable information and cover photograph used in the third edition.

And a special thank you to Australia, the home of the tea tree and of the aborigines, who are always reminding us to honor and respect our environment.

Dedication

*I dedicate this book to my children
Tamara, Kimberly, Courtney, Trent, and Terek,
whose love and friendship has sustained me,
and
to my grandchildren
Kali, Zachary, and Ashtyn,
who carry the beacon of light for Peace and
Love on the planet.*

Contents

Foreword i

Preface v

Introduction - Tea Tree Oil ix

Chapter One - History of Australian Tea Tree Oil 1
  Penfold Study 2
  Pre-World War II 3
  World War II 4

Chapter Two - Harvesting and Production 5
  Tea Tree Oil Composition 5
  Bush Oil 6
  Plantations 8
  Production 9
  Australian Tea Tree Oil Standard 10
  Specifications for the New ISO International Standard 11
  Certificate of Analysis 12

Chapter Three - First Aid Kit in a Bottle 13
  Suggested Methods of Use 13
  Eyes, Nose, Mouth and Ears 14
  Throat and Chest Conditions and the Common Cold 16
  Skin Conditions 17
  Minor Wounds, Cuts and Abrasions 20
  Feet and Nails 21
  Hair and Scalp 22
  Muscle and Joint Distress 23
  Baby Care 23
  Personal Care 25
  Precautions 26
  Patch Test 27
  Storage 27

Contents

Chapter Three (continued)
Mixing Guide 28
    Water-Soluble Concentrate 28
    Fifteen Percent Solution 28
    Twenty Percent Oil Solution 29

Chapter Four - Tea Tree Oil for Animals 31
    Tea Tree Oil for Cats and Dogs 33
        Skin Conditions 33
        Lice, Mange and Ringworm 34
        Ticks and Fleas 35
        Abscesses and Puncture Wounds................. 35
        Liniment and Insect Repellent 36
        Dental Problems 37
    Tea Tree Oil for Horses 37

Chapter Five - Testimonials 39
    Reports from Australian Practitioners 39
    Personal Testimonials 40

Chapter Six - Tea Tree Oil Products 47
    Looking Good the Healthy Way 47
        Face and Body Care 48
        Nail Care 49
        Hair Care 50
        Hair Treatments for Children................. 50
        Dental Hygiene................................ 51
        Tea Tree Oil in Aromatherapy 52
    Products Containing Tea Tree Oil 53
    The Marketplace 55

Contents

Chapter Seven - Practitioners' Guide 57
   Case Studies 57
      Pena Study: Yeast Infections 57
      H.M. Feinblatt, 1960: Boils 58
      M. Walker: Foot Problems 58
      Belaiche First Study: Thrush (Candida albicans) 59
      Belaiche Second Study: Chronic Cystitis 59
      Bacterial Vaginosis 60
      Lederle Laboratories: Acne Study 60
      Dr. Alvin Shemash: Studies of Skin Problems 61
      Podiatry Training Clinic: Geriatric Test 62
      D.S. Buck, et al: Treatment of Nail Fungus 63
      Animal Studies 64
   Clinical Research Data 65
   Toxicity Reports 70
   Safety Data 74

Appendix A - Glossary of Terms 77

Appendix B - Tea Tree Information and Specifications 81
   Weights and Measures/Conversion Table 84

Bibliography 85

Resource Guide 91

About the Author 101

Index 103

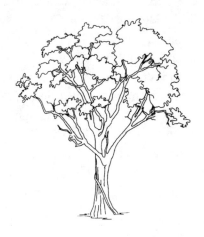

Foreword

*T*he demand for natural medicines is increasing at an unprecedented rate. All over the United States people are turning to herbs and related natural products to provide them with safe, low-cost ways to maintain and enhance health.

Herbs are big business and they have gone mainstream. They are no longer the sole province of the local natural food store or independent multi-level marketing distributor. Surveys indicate that the sale of herbs and related dietary supplements has become one of the fastest growing areas in drugstores, supermarkets and mass market retailers. One poll released in early March, 1997 by *Prevention* magazine and NBC News indicates that as many as one-third of all adult Americans are now using some type of herbal medicine. What's more, this poll determined that these adults spent an average of $54 per person on herbal products in the previous year. That tallies up to a whopping

$3.24 billion in total estimated retail herb sales—the largest estimate of the U.S. herb market to date.

Evidence of the mainstreaming of herbs is everywhere. For example, a recent edition of Dateline NBC contained a positive segment on the cardiovascular benefits of garlic while *Newsweek* carried a two-page article on the well-documented benefits of the herb St. John's wort *(Hypericum perforatum)* in treating mild to moderate cases of depression. The potential consumer draw to this issue is evidenced by the magazine's cover with following "hook" line at the top: "Natural 'Prozac': Does it Really Work?"

Consumers' demand for natural medicines has forced conventional health professionals to re-assess their long-held beliefs about their potential benefits. Many physicians and pharmacists are taking workshops or home-study courses on herbs and phytomedicines to try to catch up with their patients and customers. Harvard University has conducted three on-site conferences on "alternative medicine" in which herbal therapies were featured. In 1996 Columbia University held the first-ever week-long continuing medical education course on herbs for physicians. Other schools are developing courses on herbs for pharmacists, nurses, and dieticians.

In recent years as the herb market expanded, the message in media coverage usually dealt either with the increased consumer usage of herbs or the concerns by various health officials about their safety. However, this new publicity carries an important new theme: there is scientific and medical research that often confirms much of the traditional use of these natural medicines. The message beginning to filter into the public mind is that "Herbs really do work and there's science that proves it."

In general, people use herbs in three basic ways: First, they use herbs and medicinal plant products as substitutes for conventional, government-approved, over-the-counter non-prescription medicines to treat minor conditions or diseases. These conditions are usually self-diagnosable, self-treatable and self-limiting. That is, like a cough, cold, flu, or a muscle ache; consumers are usually capable of self-diagnosing their conditions and purchasing OTC medications to treat the problem.

Consumers also purchase herbs and related products to maintain health and wellness and to increase their overall performance, endurance and immune system functions. The popularity of tonic herbs like Asian ginseng *(Panax ginseng)* attests to this trend.

Finally, consumers use herbs as a form of preventive medicine. They believe that using herbs and other dietary supplements will help them prevent certain long-term degenerative diseases. An example is the widespread use of garlic supplements *(Allium sativum)*—still the most popular herb in mass market retail stores—which people use in the belief that garlic will help prevent or at least lower chances of developing cardiovascular disease in the long-term. There is considerable scientific research on garlic that attests to its cardiovascular benefits.

It is in this context that this book becomes a welcome addition to the explosion of information on herbs and medicinal plants. Tea tree oil *(Melaleuca alternifolia)* has become an increasingly popular ingredient in many personal and household items. With its extremely high versatility, strong germicidal activity and surprisingly low level of skin irritation, tea tree is a fairly unique substance. Scientific research and widespread consumer use in Australia and now in the U.S. strongly attests to its efficacy in treating a host of skin conditions related to bacterial and fungal infections. At the same time, the safety of tea tree oil is documented by both scientific research as well as a lack of reports of adverse reactions.

This is an important book. It presents information on tea tree oil in a concise and responsible manner. It will no doubt be useful to thousands, possibly millions, of increasingly health conscious consumers as they continue to seek authoritative information on the many applications and responsible uses of this valuable substance.

Mark Blumenthal
Founder and Executive Director, American Botanical Council
Editor, *HerbalGram*
Austin, Texas
May 1, 1997

Preface

*L*ife constantly surprises and amazes me.

In 1986 I was living in Santa Barbara, California and importing tea tree oil products into the U.S. One day Spirit tapped me on the shoulder and announced, "You are to write a book so that people will have more awareness about Australian tea tree oil." I had done many things in my life, but for me to write a book seemed out of the realm of my abilities. Spirit persisted until I said, "OK, I'll start this book, but it's going to take me a long time because I have other things I am committed to do as well." So in the evenings, when the phone stopped ringing and I could be alone, I went down to my little studio by the creek to pound away on an archaic typewriter.

My landlord at the time was a television director who was away on assignment for two years. He came to visit once and I shared with him that the only place I seemed to be able to write was in the studio. He said, "Oh, that's the only place my dad did *his* writing." His father was Jack Dewitt, journalist and author of *A Man Called Horse.*

* * * *

By the time I began to write, I had accumulated reams of information on tea tree oil. Now to sort it out and decide where to begin. Spirit led me along for a year. I didn't have a computer back then, so I found a college student from UC Santa Barbara who transcribed my notes onto disk. It was a laborious and drawn-out process, but something kept me going—some voice telling me that this was important. I was reminded that this was part of my service for mankind.

The first book, *Australian Tea Tree Oil,* turned out to be simply stated, with only 42 pages and some photographs. I had only a few hundred printed because I didn't think they would sell, and I didn't want them hanging around as a reminder of my short-lived career as an author.

One morning while sitting in my California studio, the beautiful morning light splashing subdued colors across my desk, I decided to call a distributing company in Colorado to ask if they might be interested in seeing a copy of the book. Was I surprised when the buyer said, "Yes we're interested, send us 500 books." I was still in shock after I hung up and realized that maybe this *was* a service I was providing and Spirit actually *did* assist me in this process. Quickly, I ordered a printing of 3,000 books, having more faith now that these books would be sold. They were; and after seven years and two more books on tea tree oil, the books continue to sell—over 500,000 copies to date, translated into five languages—further confirmation that Spirit was indeed guiding me in the right direction.

* * * *

My introduction to tea tree oil began in 1985, on a blind date orchestrated by my youngest daughter and her best friend. The man they chose was her friend's father. I remember my daughter saying that this man was special and so like me in many ways—into holistic health, meditation, and organic food. I showed up at his place holding a bouquet of flowers and a bottle of wine. When he opened the door, he looked very surprised. He later shared with me that he had never received flowers from a woman before, and the surprise was pleasant. I found out his passion was working with plants and flowers, and he owned a rather large nursery.

He took me out to his organic vegetable garden, and it was there that I stepped into a fire ant hill. We immediately applied tea tree oil to take away the sting. I had never heard of this stuff with the peculiar odor. Now twelve years have passed and not a day goes by that I don't use the oil in some way, whether it's brushing my teeth or applying it to my skin. My blind date turned out to be my working and living partner until 1990.

* * * *

I am eternally grateful for my journey, though it hasn't always been a bed of roses. My parents died within two months of each other when I was 25. I managed through two marriages and divorces, and raised five children. One day I realized that with all our moving around, I had lived in 14 states. There were times I severely doubted myself and went into depression, feeling as though my skin had been turned inside out, and I had no idea what the next step would be. When I moved back to Colorado, I realized that it was time to surrender—to let go of all my preconceived notions that had served me well up to now (I fought *that* one with as much intensity as an Aries could muster). Finally one day I knelt down, cried, threw my hands up to the heavens and boomed, "OK, God, I surrender to You. Help me!"

My days since then have been simply startling. I ask for guidance, check in as to where I am to be, what I am to do, and then let go. I am on a great adventure and so thankful to experience everyone and everything that touches me. Now Spirit has again tapped me on the shoulder and said, "One more time, write an updated book on tea tree oil. It's time."

My purpose in writing the guide six years ago was to share the wonderful story of Australian tea tree oil with people who were looking for alternative medicines. That purpose hasn't changed. If anything, natural medicine is becoming more mainstream. The baby-boomers now make up a large portion of consumers in the natural products industry. Sales of herbs in natural health food stores and chain stores in this country rose over 20% between 1994 and 1996.

How does tea tree oil fit in to this picture? Airborne viruses and immune deficiency disorders are becoming commonplace in our society, and traditional allopathic medicine doesn't seem to have the capability to control, let alone cure, these chronic illnesses. Herbs and oils such as tea tree may be the solution for the future.

Cynthia Olsen
May, 1997

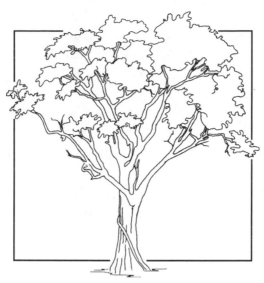

Introduction
Tea Tree Oil

*A*n estimated sixty million years ago, as the continents of earth continued to shift and change shape, an immense land mass measuring more than three million square miles gradually separated from the Asian mainland and formed the largest island on earth—*Australia.*

"The Lucky Country," "The Quiet Continent," "Last of Lands," "New Australia," and "New Holland" are just a few of the names used by seventeenth-century Dutch explorers to describe this land. Australia was called "upside down," because, unlike the United States or Europe, southern Australia faces toward Antarctica and is relatively cool; by contrast, the northern region is near the equator, warm and tropical, and supports a rich diversity of life ranging from the mountains to the plains, vast deserts of the outback to peaceful lagoons, lush rain forests to the Great Barrier Reef.

Foremost among the rare and unusual trees growing along Australia's east coast, in the swampy, low-lying lands of New South Wales, is the *Melaleuca alternifolia* or "Tea Tree," from which comes the oil with the amazing healing and therapeutic properties.

"I think it [tea tree oil] is a great natural resource for Australia. Australia has a real treasure there; particularly in this century in which we're living, where there's a renewed outbreak of infectious diseases and pollution."

Dr. Paul Belaiche,
Chief of Phytotherapy Department,
Faculty of Medicine,
University of Paris, Paris, France

The folklore surrounding the aborigines of the Australian outback is filled with mystique about their use of nature's gifts as medicine. The story goes that the Bundjalung aborigines living in the bush country would pick tea tree leaves, which were coated with the wondrous oil, and rub the leaf on their skin to alleviate cuts, bites, burns, and other skin ailments. They ground the leaves into a fine paste for dressing wounds, and crushed the leaves to use as an insect repellent. The aborigines also sought lakes and pools of bronze-colored water and sat in these pools to heal their sore and infected bodies. These pools were surrounded by tea trees; their bronze color came from the oil dripping from the tea tree leaves into the water.

Outside Australia, it has been known for nearly 100 years that tea tree oil is a powerful antiseptic, bactericide, and fungicide. Many studies on the increased uses for tea tree oil have taken place in the last five years. Tea tree oil has been studied to treat acne, burns, thrush (yeast), candida, and fungal infections. These studies are discussed in Chapter Seven, the Practitioners' Guide.

There are various grades of tea tree oil, among them pharmaceutical grade (for human and animal use), usually containing at least 35% terpinen-4-ol and less than 5% cineole; standard grade, which contains between 30-35% terpinen-4-ol and as much as 8% cineole; and industrial grade for commercial use. Both standard and industrial grades are used for disinfectants, mold and fungus killers, floor detergents, and in air conditioning and venting systems.

Tea tree oil is a renewable resource; it is non-corrosive, non-staining, economical, easy to use, and may be added to a wide variety of products. When dissolved in water, it maintains its clear properties. Tea tree oil is already being used in major body care products sold in department stores and drugstores throughout the U.S. More information on these uses appear in Chapter Six, "Tea Tree Oil Products."

* * * *

Tea tree oil stands out among natural herbal remedies and has proven time and time again that it is truly a *first aid kit in a bottle.*

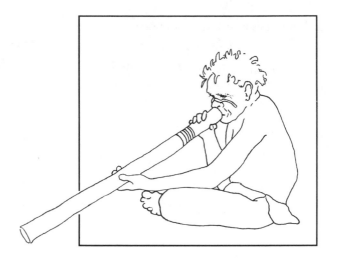

Chapter One

History of Australian Tea Tree Oil

*I*n 1770, Captain James Cook (at that time a lieutenant) of the British Royal Navy disembarked from the H.M.S. *Endeavour* at Botany Bay, Australia—near the eventual site of Sydney. Captain Cook was accompanied by Joseph Banks, a young botanist (later Sir Joseph, president of the Royal Society for 40 years). Banks was a wealthy landowner who traveled with four servants and two large dogs. Banks paid the expenses for all of the scientists aboard the *Endeavour*. His presence on the expedition enhanced the scientific scope of Cook's voyage and paved the way for other scientists to participate in future expeditions—perhaps even Darwin's exploration aboard the ship *Beagle* sixty years later.

Cook's party came across the indigenous people, "poor Stone Age fellows," whom he described as shy but fearless, and adept at throwing spears 40-50 feet. Cook noted: "...the aborigines kept out of the way, except to go fishing in their primitive canoes, the worst I think I ever saw." He said of them: "In reality they are far more happier [sic] than we Europeans...they live in a Tranquility which is not disturbed by the Inequality of Condition; the Earth and sea of their own accord furnishes them with all the things necessary for life..."

"...We at first made it <some beer> of a decoction of the spruce leaves; but finding that this alone made the beer too astringent, we afterwards mixed it with an equal quantity of the tea plant (a name it obtained in my former voyage from our using it as tea then, as we also did now) which partly destroyed the astringency of the other, and made the beer exceedingly palatable, and esteemed by everyone on board."

Captain Cook's account of his second voyage, "A Voyage Towards the South Pole," *National Geographic* (Vol. 1, p. 99, 1977)

From Botany Bay the party continued its way north through the coastal region of New South Wales, where they came upon groves of trees thick with sticky, aromatic leaves that, when boiled, rendered a spicy tea. Joseph Banks collected samples of the leaves and brought them back to England for further study. These early explorers could not have known that 150 years later, *Melaleuca alternifolia*, or "Tea Trees" as they were called by Captain Cook, would be used as a medicinal agent for cuts, burns, bites, and a host of skin ailments.

Penfold Study

In 1923, Dr. A.R. Penfold, curator and chemist at the Government Museum of Technology and Applied Sciences in Sydney, conducted a study of the leaves of the "tea tree." Dr. Penfold discovered their essential oils to be thirteen times stronger as an antiseptic bactericide than carbolic acid, considered the universal standard in the early 1900's. In 1925 Penfold announced his findings before the Royal Society of New South Wales and England.

Dr. Penfold noted: "Melaleuca alternifolia is quite common, and exists in very large areas in the North Coast district of New South Wales. It yields 1.8% of an oil of pale lemon tint, with a pleasant terpenic myristic odor. This is prepared on a commercial scale, and is particularly recommended as a non-poisonous non-irritant antiseptic and disinfectant of unusual strength, the Rideal-Walker coefficient being 11. The oil contains 50-60% of terpenes (pinenes, terpinene and cymene), from 6-8% of cineole (accounting for the camphoraceous odor) and an alcohol terpineol, which supplies the pleasant nutmeg-like odor, also small amounts of sesquiterpenes and their corresponding alcohols... The valuable antiseptic properties of the oil and its spicy flavoring note should provide useful in dentifrices and mouthwashes."

In the 1930's tea tree oil was used as an antiseptic in dressing wounds, and was useful in oral hygiene. In a hand soap it was found to be 60 times more effective than other disinfectants against typhoid bacilli.

Pre-World War II

Research continued, and by 1930 the editors of the *Medical Journal of Australia* reported that applying tea tree oil to pus-filled infections dissolved the pus and left the surface of infected wounds clean and without apparent irritation to healthy tissues. The article also stated that application of tea tree oil on infected nail beds eradicated the damage within one week. It was also noted that a few drops of oil in a tumbler of warm water, as a gargle, helped to soothe sore throats. In 1933, publications such as the *Australian Journal of Pharmacy, The Journal of the National Medical Association (U.S.A.)* and the *British Medical Journal*, indicated that the oil is a powerful disinfectant, non-poisonous and non-irritating, and that it has been used successfully in a very wide range of septic conditions. Research showed that tea tree oil was successfully administered around the world for throat and mouth conditions, for gynecological conditions, and in dental treatment for pyorrhea and gingivitis. It also had an extraordinary effect on a variety of skin fungi including candida, tinea, and perionychia.

Even before World War II, there were scientific claims about this unique oil. In 1936, *The Medical Journal of Australia* reported that tea tree oil successfully treated diabetic gangrene. Also, in 1936 a magazine called *Poultry* announced that tea tree oil (known at that time as

Ti-Trol) prevented cannibalism in poultry. When the Ti-Trol was applied to chickens, the odor of the oil kept the chickens from pecking at one another. In 1937 it was noted that in the presence of blood, pus, and other matter, the oil's antiseptic features were increased 10-12%.

World War II

During World War II, tea tree oil was considered to be such a necessary commodity that cutters and producers were exempted from war service until sufficient reserves of the oil had been accumulated to permit its standard issue in first aid kits for the Army and Naval units in the tropical regions. Large quantities of Melaleuca alternifolia oil were blended with machine cutting oils, to kill bacteria and reduce infections from skin injuries, especially abrasions to the hands caused by metal filings and turnings. Eventually demand exceeded supply and synthetic alternatives were developed.

About this time, synthetic drugs gained popularity as miracle drugs and eventually pushed tea tree oil into the shadows. But with the arrival of the 1960's and "flower power," a new awareness took hold throughout the West. Toxic substances and synthetic medicine began to lose favor as a new generation turned to natural medicines. By the 1970's tea tree oil was rediscovered.

"We have only partially tapped the domestic market, let alone the world market. Just consider if every Chinese soldier carried 25 ml [less than 1 oz.] of tea tree oil, all his needs of his first aid kit, what an amount that would require."

Brian Fletcher
ABC Radio Australia, 1986.

In the 1980's, an optometrist named Brian Fletcher was working to clone the Melaleuca alternifolia tree with the most excellent properties. Fletcher died in an accident in 1990; however, the University of New England was provided a federal government grant to implement the cloning project.

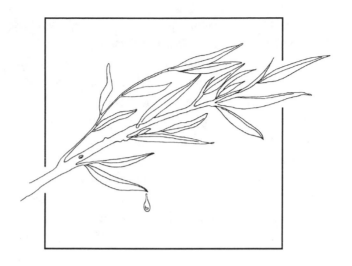

Chapter Two

Harvesting and Production

$\mathcal{T}$ea Tree Oil Composition

The Melaleuca alternifolia is a narrow-leafed paper bark tree twenty feet in height. Its oil is made up of almost 100 compounds, 21 of which have yet to be identified.[1] Some of these compounds, such as *viridflorene,* had never been found in nature, so names had to be created. It appears that all compounds work in synergy to produce an essential oil with antiseptic and fungicidal properties. The oil color may vary from colorless to pale yellow. The aroma is pungent and resembles eucalyptus. The bush oil (oil from trees found in their natural habitat) appears to have a heartier aroma than plantation oil. Sometimes if the oil is too pungent it may indicate an inferior grade.

---

[1]*Journal of the American Academy of Dermatology,* Vol. 30, No. 3, March 1994

Two of the chemical compounds that are tested from batch to batch are cineole and terpinen-4-ol. Both of these ingredients need to meet certain percentages according to the Australian standard. (Refer to the standard at the end of this chapter.) If cineole is above 15%, it will become caustic to the skin. Cineole should be 5% or less, and terpinen-4-ol should be above 30%; in fact, the higher the concentration of terpinen-4-ol the better, since this compound is known to contain healing and antiseptic properties.

Even though tea trees have been studied since 1923, there is much more to be discovered about them. For instance, the trees grow in a specific region of New South Wales and yet the oil, upon testing, may vary from batch to batch and tree to tree. Even the tried and true method of steam distilling the oil may affect and change the consistency of the compounds.

Tea trees have not always been looked upon as a wonder of nature; in fact, for years Australian farmers considered them a nuisance. The farmers wanted to clear the trees off their land so they could raise cattle, sugar cane, and tobacco; however, tea trees have tenacious root systems that go quite deep. Yanking out a tree is not an easy task and if any roots are left intact, the tree will surface again quickly.

Bush Oil

The natural habitat of Melaleuca alternifolia is the swampy, low-lying land around the Clarence and Richmond River systems where a multitude of established trees thrive. There are over 300 varieties of Melaleuca; however only one, the Melaleuca alternifolia, contains great amounts of antiseptic and fungicidal qualities.

Currently, the only area where Melaleuca alternifolia grows in its natural state is in the northeastern region of New South Wales. The consistency of the oil varies from tree to tree. However, the trees that grow in the Clarence-Richmond River areas appear to contain higher levels of terpinen-4-ol and lower levels of cineole, which produces an ideal combination for healing purposes.

The harvesting and processing of "bush oil" began in the 1920's. For many years, a score of small producers would venture into the area with skilled leaf cutters and harvest the branches of the trees. The Melaleuca alternifolia thrives in remote "flood-prone" wetlands; therefore, harvesting the leaves is extremely laborious. In the early days of bush oil production, the 'cutters' were faced with hordes of wasps and hundreds of snakes which hunted for frogs around the swamps. One distiller was badly burned on his arms, legs, back, and buttocks when his still exploded. He spent three weeks in a hospital and emerged with little or no scarring, which he claimed was because it was the tea tree steam that burned him and the tea tree steam that cured him!

"You had to be hardy to do the work. Sometimes you'd be struggling through water and step in a hole and find yourself up to your waist in it. You couldn't work without boots, you might tread on a snake. I've done that, too. One of the things you have to contend with is the smoke from the burning of the 'spent leaf.' You're left with a pile of ash—it's good fertilizer; it has a pungent smell, not terribly pleasant. If the leaf's a bit wet there'll be a very dense cloud of smoke. People always knew where you were."

Artie Ford[2]

The cutters used lightweight, razor-sharp machetes to cut the suckers off the stumps before stripping each branch with a cane knife. The dense brush has prevented all attempts at mechanized harvesting where even four-wheel drive vehicles frequently get trapped in the mud.

In spite of these obstacles, experienced cutters work very quickly, using a simple technique of holding branches upside down with one hand while cutting with the other. This method of harvesting prevents any damage to the trees or the surrounding ecosystem. In fact, the growth of the tree seems to be stimulated by regular cropping. Some of the trees along the Bungawalbyn Creek have been harvested for over 60 years and are healthy and hardy. Experienced cutters can harvest a ton of leaves in a day's work, which yields ten liters of oil.

---

[2] Marie Newman, *Australia's Own Tea Tree Oil*, Mid-Richmond Historical Society, Coraki, NSW, Australia, 1992.

Once the leaves are pruned, they are brought to a steam distiller unit, also called a "bush still." The harvested leaf is placed in racks inside the steamer. The still is heated by burning wood; once the water boils to a certain temperature, the steam passes through the leaves and the capillaries burst, releasing the essential oil which passes to a collection tank. The oil floats to the top where it is filtered and poured into containers to be shipped to the marketplace.

The modern method of distillation, used on many plantations, is to generate the steam in a separate boiler, vs. the bush method where the leaf material sits above the boiling water. The steam from the boiler is then injected into a distillation pot. In this method, it takes only two to three hours for the steam to pass through the leaf material, produce the oil, condense and separate it. The discarded leaf is often used as mulch in the fields.

* * * *

Are the 'bush days' gone in New South Wales? Have plantations replaced the good old methods of distilling in the back country? Bush oil is still produced, but it is under threat from environmentalists, particularly where it occurs in the state forests. Production and plantations have grown dramatically in the last several years. Even Crocodile Dundee has gotten into the tea tree business.

Plantations

In the past, most production of tea tree oil has been derived from natural stands of trees; however, besides being labor-intensive due to the inaccessibility of the trees, production is limited and adverse weather can affect the operation.

With the increasing interest in tea tree oil, growers and producers are beginning to plan ahead so that supply will be able to keep up with world-wide demand. Thus, tea tree plantations began to appear in the mid-eighties and are now springing up all around New South Wales. Plantations now account for the bulk of tea tree oil production. Although operating costs can be high, the agricultural system is efficient enough to keep production costs down. To increase production, plantations have established nutrition systems which may include fertilizing as well as control of weeds, pests, and diseases. It is always good to ask if oils are produced from organic farms; the largest plantation in New South Wales, Main Camp (Bungawalbyn Valley), is an organic farm which accounts for half of the world's production of tea tree oil.

Because tea tree seeds are extremely small, it is more economical to establish seedlings in trays. Transplanted seedlings can produce thirty to forty thousand plants per hectare (approximately 2½ acres), with annual yields of 150 to 200 kg. per hectare. Sandy loam or light-textured soil appears to be preferable for growing tea trees; planting in valleys with good irrigation is important as well. Wind dries the limbs, so sheltering the plant helps to reduce damage. Since tea trees require moisture, plantations have had to rely on irrigation. Tea trees tolerate some flooding, although full immersion may kill trees if they are flooded for more than a week.

In the spring, tea trees produce a white bloom; if harvested after the flowering, a higher yield and better quality oil can be expected. Summer is the season for production of the oil, which, in Australia, is December through May. The trees grow rapidly during the hot summer months and appear to slow their growth in the winter.

Production

In the 1980's, the annual production of tea tree oil amounted to 15 to 20 tons. With more plantations appearing, the production has now increased to approximately 300 tons annually. That number could conceivably rise to 700 tons within the next several years. Anywhere from 60 to 100 tons of oil are currently being imported into North America, including bulk oil and the oil sold to companies to add to their product lines. Currently the U.S. Department of Commerce does not assess a duty on imported tea tree oil, but may do so when the import amount rises above $10 million.

Approximately 50 companies carry tea tree oil products in their lines. Most oil, however, is purchased by a few large companies to include in their products and resell to other companies. There is also increasing interest from Europe, China, and India to purchase the oil in bulk amounts.

In the U.S., multi-level companies are doing a great business. One in particular, which manufactures over sixty tea tree products, had a revenue of $100 million in 1995.

Given the increased interest in the tea tree industry, there is a strong indication that tea tree oil could develop into an industry worth $20 to $25 million within the next ten years. This amount reflects products containing tea tree oil (approximately 30% of total tea tree oil production), not in bulk oil sales. The price of bulk oil also may fluctuate due to the changes in the supply and demand of the product. Tea tree oil currently sells for around $45-50 kg. ($20-22/lb.). Organic oil may be $4-5/lb. higher.

Australian Tea Tree Oil Standard

There have been three standards established for Australian tea tree oil; the first, AS 175-1967, was specifically for Melaleuca alternifolia and clearly designated Melaleuca alternifolia as being the oil for therapeutic uses.

In the 1980's, The Australian Tea Tree Industry Association (ATTIA), made up of Australian growers, buyers, and exporters, was formed to establish guidelines for the industry. These guidelines included minimum percentages for terpinen-4-ol and maximum percentages for cineole. The standard AS 2782-1985 was adopted in 1985, assuring that the oil would contain at least 30% terpinen-4-ol, and a maximum of 15% cineole. This standard permitted blending of other tea tree oils, as long as these percentages were met.

Due to the increased awareness of Melaleuca alternifolia in the world marketplace, the temptation was great to dilute Melaleuca alternifolia oil with other oils or to use a tea tree oil other than Melaleuca alternifolia. No clinical data has been produced to support the efficacy of a blended oil. Since tea tree compounds are so unique, blending other types of tea trees (over 300 varieties) or blending other types of oils may affect the careful balance that nature has provided.

A new Australian standard (ISO 4730) has been officially adopted by the International Standards Organization, and will replace standard AS 2782-1985 this year. Specifications for the new standard are listed below.

Specifications for the New ISO International Standard

ISO Standard 4730 states that tea tree oil should be extracted from the *Melaleuca alternifolia, Melaleuca linafolia,* or *Melaleuca dissitifolia* species of the Myrtaceae family. Other tea tree species, including Cajuput *(Melaleuca Cajuputi),* New Zealand Manuka *(Leptospermum scoparium),* New Zealand Ti-Tree *(Cordyline australis),* and Kanuka *(Leptospermum ericoides)* are not highly regarded, as they do not contain the same anti-microbial benefits, nor have they been in use for nearly a century as has Melaleuca alternifolia.

See page 12 for a certificate of analysis of Main Camp pharmaceutical grade oil, with specifications relevant to the new ISO Standard.

* * * *

It is important for distributors and consumers to be certain that the tea tree oil they sell or use is authentic pharmaceutical grade tea tree oil that falls into the guidelines of the new Australian standard. It may be wise to ask the importer to send a copy of testing done on the particular batch of oil being purchased.

The American Tea Tree Association (ATTA) helps to monitor the quality and purity of oil imported into this country. According to Martha Smith, treasurer of ATTA, under FDA labeling regulations, a synthetic oil could not be labeled as pure tea tree oil. Pure tea tree oil can be blended from different batches, however. Testing on questionable oil has identified some 'bogus' oil, and suppliers of that oil have been confronted within the industry. A gas chromatograph will reveal the components of oil.

NSW Agriculture
Registered T.G.A. Laboratory
License No. 55187

Certificate of Analysis

Sample: Australian Plantations
Date: July 17, 1997
Batch No.:   97/03
Laboratory Ref: 97-761

Analytical Results

1. **Gas Chromatographic Analysis**

Test	Specifications	Results
α-pinene	1.0 - 6.0%	2.4
Sabinene	trace - 3.5%	0.4
α-terpinene	5.0 - 13.0%	10.0
Limonene	0.5 - 4.0%	0.9
ρ-cymene	0.5 - 12.0%	1.8
1,8 cineole	Maximum 15%	2.0
γ-terpinine	10.0% - 28.0%	21.5
Terpinolene	1.5% - 5.0%	3.5
Terpinen 4-ol	Minimum 30%	41.6
α-terpineol	1.5% - 8.0%	3.1
Aromadendrene	trace - 7.0%	1.1
Ledene	0.5 - 6.5%	0.9
δ-cadinene	trace - 8.0%	1.0
Globulol	trace - 3.0%	0.5
Viridiflorol	trace - 1.5%	0.2

	Client Results	ISO RANGE
2. **Relative Density (20°C)**	0.894	0.885 - 0.906
3. **Refractive Index (20°C)**	1.477	1.475 - 1.482
4. **Optical Rotation (20°C)**	9.6	+5° - +15°
5. **Solubility in 85% (v/v) Ethanol (20°C)**	0.9 ml	Less than 2 ml

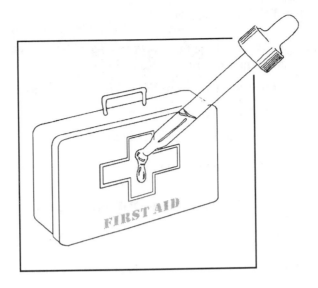

Chapter Three

First Aid Kit in a Bottle

*T*ea tree oil is fast becoming a natural first aid for American families. Throughout the twentieth century clinical data has been collected, providing information on the uses of tea tree oil in hospitals (as an antiseptic), for dental problems, yeast infections, chronic cystitis, foot problems, acne, fungus, candida, and many other conditions.

This chapter is intended as an easy reference guide for the most common uses of tea tree oil.

Suggested Methods of Use

A: Mix one part pure tea tree oil with ten parts of a quality cold-pressed oil such as olive, almond, apricot kernel, avocado, etc.

B: Add ten or so drops of pure tea tree oil to a bowl of hot water, bath water, humidifier, or vaporizer.

C: Add ten drops of pure tea tree oil to an 8 oz. quantity of natural (non-detergent) shampoo or conditioner.

D.   Add five to ten drops to 'boost' tea tree creams or lotions.

E: Use undiluted tea tree oil.

F: Add three to five drops to one cup water.

See page 28 for instructions on making other tea tree solutions.

Eyes, Nose, Mouth and Ears

Problem	Method	Application
Blocked Nasal or Sinus Passages	B	heat a pot of solution on the stove. Let it come to a boil and, tenting your face with a towel, lean over and allow the steam to fill your face and inhale gently. *Do not get too close to the steam.* You can also sprinkle several drops of the oil onto a hot, wet cloth and place over nose for five minutes.
Canker Sores	E	gently apply a few drops of oil directly to infected area with cotton swab, twice daily. Also add three drops to a tumbler of water, swish around mouth. Do not swallow.
Chapped Lips		apply a tea tree lip balm.
Cold Sores Mouth Ulcers	E	gently apply a few drops of oil directly to infected area with cotton swab, twice daily. To help prevent breakout, apply at onset.
Earaches		warm a quarter cup of olive oil with five drops of tea tree oil, drop a small amount into ear, pack ear loosely with a small cotton ball to allow oil to remain in ear; repeat as necessary.

Eyes, Nose, Mouth and Ears (continued)

Problem	Method	Application
Gingivitis	E/F	rub swollen and sore area of gum with pure tea tree oil. Add three to five drops of oil to small glass of water, swish around mouth twice daily.
Nasal Ulcers	E	dab two to three drops of the oil directly on to affected area; apply pure tea tree oil with a cotton swab.
Sore gums, bad breath, plaque	F/E	add three to five drops to water and use as a mouthwash twice daily. Add a few drops to toothpaste. Also rub a few drops of the pure oil into the gums and massage. Keep toothbrush germ-free by soaking in a dilute solution of tea tree oil (5 to 10 drops in 1/2 cup water) for 10 minutes, then rinse. Use tea tree floss.
Styes	B	place face over a bowl of hot water in which five drops of tea tree oil have been added; steam for five minutes. It is advisable not to apply oil directly to the eye area, as it will sting and may become quite irritated.
Toothache	F/E	rinse teeth with gargle mixture; apply a few drops tea tree oil directly onto infected tooth.

Throat and Chest Conditions and the Common Cold

Problem	Method	Application
Bronchial Congestion	E	steam chest with a mixture of five drops of pure oil on a warm, wet cloth applied to chest.
Congestion/Coughs	B/E	add ten drops pure oil to steam bath or vaporizer-inhale. Rub pure oil into chest and back. Sprinkle a few drops on pillow before sleeping.
Emphysema	B/E	add pure oil to vaporizer or pot of steaming water-inhale vapors. Follow directions for bronchial congestion.
Head Cold	B/E	gently inhale steam from vaporizer or hot water. At night, use steam vaporizer with ten drops of oil. Rub a few drops on nose and forehead.
Sore Throat	F	add five drops of pure oil to a cup of warm water and gargle two to three times a day. Use tea tree lozenges.
Thrush	F	follow instructions for sore throat.

"I have found in my own personal experience that the tea tree oil is a fantastic curative for most any kind of dermatological problems including nasal ulcer, athlete's foot, and rashes of all kinds."

William L. Mayo, Ph. D., President
American Society for Environmental Education

Skin Conditions

Problem	Method	Application
Acne	E	apply three drops of oil to infected area twice daily, or combine one oz. of tea tree oil with 10 oz. water or a mixture of witch hazel and rosewater; apply mixture to area twice daily. Add oil to facewash and use moisturizing cream. Use tea tree soaps and creams.
Boils	E	apply several drops of pure oil three times daily.
Burns (minor)	E	immediately flush area with ice water for one to two minutes. Alternate application of 100% tea tree oil with ice water for up to one hour, depending on severity of burn. Continue to massage tea tree oil into burn twice daily for three to four days. Tea tree oil may be applied to blistered burns to help minimize blistering and prevent infection. Make a burn salve of 5 oz. raw, unpasteurized honey mixed with 1 oz. tea tree oil and 1 teaspoon grapefruit seed extract.[3]
Dermatitis	A	massage several drops of mixture into area. To help moisturize the skin, massage tea tree cream into areas that have been exposed to water. Try a tea tree soap as well.
Eczema	E	make sure skin is dry and apply tea tree oil to affected area. A tea tree lotion, cream or soap would also be helpful.

[3]Puotinen, C.J. *Nature's Antiseptics: Tea Tree Oil and Grapefruit Seed Extract.* New Canaan, CT; Keats Publishing, Inc., 1997.

Skin Conditions (continued)

Problem	Method	Application
Hives	E	massage oil into affected area. Tea tree lotion can also be used.
Insect Bites and Stings	E/A	apply oil to affected area. For larger areas, combine five drops of tea tree oil with a cold-pressed oil such as almond, apricot kernel or avocado. Use tea tree lotions, available in health and body care stores. As an insect repellant, apply oil to exposed skin.
Leeches/Ticks	E	apply a drop or two of pure oil to kill parasite; when leech falls off, apply oil again; for ticks, gently remove tick with tweezers, then apply full strength tea tree oil to area.
Leg Ulcers	E	massage a few drops pure oil into affected area two to three times daily. If irritation occurs, discontinue use of pure oil and use tea tree lotion or cream instead.
Poison Oak and Poison Ivy	E/A	twice daily, massage affected area with tea tree oil or mixture of tea tree oil and cold-pressed oil. Apply tea tree oil ointment or lotion as well.
Psoriasis	E	apply to affected area and follow instructions for dermatitis and eczema.
Rashes	A/E	apply the oil or use a tea tree lotion; a tea tree soap may prove useful as well.

Skin Conditions (continued)

Problem	Method	Application
Ringworm	E	apply pure oil to area. Repeat twice daily.
Sandfleas/Stings	E/A	apply several drops of oil on affected area; use tea tree oil mixture or cream to treat larger areas.
Shingles	A	warm mixture and apply to painful area two to three times daily until pain subsides.
Sore Nipples		if nipples are sore, dry, or cracked, massage a small amount of tea tree lotion onto the area.
Sunburn	A/E	to bring relief and prevent blistering, use a tea tree cream and/or mix with oil as in method A. Apply twice daily. For severe cases of sunburn, apply pure oil.
Tropical Ulcers, Plantar Warts, Coral Cuts	E	dab some oil on affected area three times per day.
Warts	E	use pure oil until wart dries. May take several weeks depending on condition.

"Research has shown that tea tree oil is four to five times stronger than the usual household disinfectants (i.e., hydrogen peroxide), and yet it stings far less when applied to minor abrasions."

Robert Tisserand
*The International Journal
of Aromatherapy*, February 1988

Minor Wounds, Cuts and Abrasions

Problem	Method	Application
Abrasions	E	clean area well and follow instruction for cuts.
After Shave	E	for men, apply a few drops of oil or tea tree cream. Redness usually subsides within a day. Tea tree oil can be applied onto razor blade when shaving to help cut down on nicks. Apply a few drops of the pure oil or tea tree cream as an aftershave to act as an antiseptic and eliminate ingrown hairs.
Cuts	E	wash area with tea tree soap; apply a few drops of pure oil and tea tree lotion.
Dog Bites	E/F	flush bite with tea tree solution; cleanse with soap and water and apply tea tree oil full strength or diluted. Repeat three times daily for several days. Seek medical attention immediately if you cannot verify whether animal has had rabies vaccination, or if condition worsens.

Feet and Nails

Problem	Method	Application
Athlete's Foot *(tinea)*	E/A/F	wash feet with an anti-fungal soap and dry thoroughly. Apply pure tea tree oil (or oil mixed with olive oil) onto and between toes. A solution of tea tree oil and water may be used to disinfect socks.
Corns and Callouses	A	apply a mixture of several drops of tea tree oil and olive oil and massage into the area well. A foot soak is useful, adding five drops of tea tree into a small amount of almond or olive oil and soaking for five minutes.
Foot Odor	B/E	add five to ten drops of pure oil to warm bath water, or rub oil directly into feet.
Nail Infection *(perionychia)*	A	remove polish, smooth nail surface, shape nails. Warm a tea tree hand and body lotion or pure oil blended into olive or almond oil. Soak for five minutes. Massage lotion around nailbeds twice daily until infection clears.
Plantar Warts	A	follow instructions for corns/callouses.

"...tea tree oil is the best treatment I know for fungal infections of the skin (athlete's foot, ringworm, jock itch). It will also clear up fungal infections of the toenails and fingernails, a condition notoriously resistant to treatment, even by strong systemic antibiotics. You just paint the oil on affected areas two or three times a day."

Andrew Weil, M.D.
Natural Health, Natural Medicine

Hair and Scalp

Problem	Method	Application
Dandruff	C	use a tea tree oil shampoo or shampoo mixture; use daily or alternate with another natural shampoo. Leave on for a minute or so before rinsing. Rub a few drops of the oil directly into the scalp to help unblock hair follicles.
Dry Hair	C/E	shampoo daily or during usual routine; work up rich lather with small amount of shampoo mixture. Rinse and shampoo again. You can also apply five to ten drops of oil directly onto hair strands or massage into scalp.
Head Lice (*pediculus humans capitis*)	D/C	apply a tea tree oil shampoo boosted with ten additional drops of pure tea tree oil. Leave on ten minutes; rinse. Repeat once or twice a week. Soak combs, brushes, and other contaminated material in a tea tree oil solution to guard again continued infection.
Itchy Scalp	E/C	use tea tree oil shampoo or a few drops of tea tree oil directly on scalp.
Oily Hair	C/E	shampoo daily. A few drops of tea tree oil rubbed into the scalp will also aid oily scalp, as well as dry and itchy scalp and dandruff.
Thinning Hair	E/C	use a tea tree oil shampoo or mix five to ten drops of oil into your regular shampoo; use daily or alternate with another natural shampoo. Rub a few drops of the oil directly into the scalp to help unblock hair follicles.

Muscle and Joint Distress

Problem	Method	Application
Arthritis	A	warm tea tree mixture and massage into painful joints.
Bruises	E/D	apply pure oil directly to affected area, massage in well twice daily; or mix four parts *arnica Montana* tincture with one part tea tree oil– apply every few hours for two or three days, as needed.
Muscle Aches	E/A/B	massage pure oil into area or add five drops to warm almond oil; massage in well. Bathe in warm water adding ten drops of pure oil.
Sprains	A	massage into damaged area, using same mixture as for shingles; add ten drops of tea tree oil to bathwater and soak.

Baby Care

It is important to remember that babies have very sensitive skin. It is best to mix the oil with a quality cold-pressed oil. Look for companies who carry tea tree baby care products.

Problem	Method	Application
Breast Feeding	E	if breasts are sore, dry, or cracked, massage a small amount of tea tree lotion onto the area.
Colds	B	add ten drops of pure oil to a bowl of hot water or vaporizer, leave vaporizer in baby's area overnight (out of reach) or whenever indicated. A small handkerchief sprinkled with tea tree under child's pillow may help as well.

Baby Care (continued)

Problem	Method	Application
Cradle Cap	A/C	mix five drops of pure oil with olive oil, rub into scalp, leave for five minutes, wash and rinse. Use a tea tree oil shampoo mixture being very careful to keep out of child's eyes.
Diaper Cleanser		add twenty drops of pure oil or a water miscible formula to each gallon of water. Stir and soak diapers overnight.
Diaper Rash		*do not apply pure tea tree oil to a baby's bottom.* Use a tea tree oil cream. Apply whenever you change the diaper until redness subsides.
Ear Infections		warm five to ten drops of pure oil mixed with a teaspoon of almond or olive oil. Trickle a small amount in ear. Apply as needed.
Insect Bites	A	dab a few drops of mixture directly onto bite. Massage tea tree lotion into affected areas as well.
Room Deodorizer and Disinfectant	B/E	if you have a diffuser, add a few drops of tea tree oil to it to freshen and clean the baby's area. A humidifier or vaporizer will work as well; adding five to ten drops of oil to the water will add a wonderful mist to the baby's room.
Skin Rashes	E/A	dab a few drops directly onto area. *Do not use pure oil for larger areas;* tea tree cream or lotion is recommended.

Personal Care

Problem	Method	Application
Bikini Waxing	E	before waxing, apply three to five drops of pure oil on area; allow to dry. After treatment, apply oil again and follow up with tea tree lotion; repeat two times same day. Redness and swelling should subside within twenty-four hours. Helps to eliminate ingrown hairs.
Hemorrhoids	E/B	apply several drops of pure oil directly onto affected area; soak in tub using ten drops of oil in tub water. Also may use tea tree ointment or cream on area. For extreme swelling, a tea tree oil suppository may be used.
Herpes Lesions	E/A	apply pure tea tree oil, just a few drops onto affected area; oil may be mixed with a vitamin E oil. Apply twice daily. If irritation occurs, discontinue use.
Ovarian Cysts		if possible, obtain tea tree oil suppositories through your health store; insert. The suppository will melt and help to reduce the cysts. If suppositories are not available, use a tea tree oil saturated tampon, similar to directions for vaginal infections. If symptoms don't change, consult your physician.
Vaginal Cleansing	B	douche with eight to ten drops of pure tea tree oil mixed into one pint of distilled or purified water. Ten drops of pure oil may be added to a warm tub of water for your bath; soak for twenty minutes.

Personal Care (continued)

Problem	Method	Application
Vaginal Infection (yeast infections)	B/E	douche with vaginal formula (see vaginal cleansing). Treatment can be done daily until symptoms subside or disappear. In between douching, saturate a tampon or a sea sponge (see Testimonials, page 44) with several drops of tea tree oil and insert. Leave in twenty-four hours. A slight cooling sensation may be felt.

If any of the previous conditions persist following recommended treatment, discontinue and consult a physician.

Please read the precaution section below.

Precautions

1. Avoid contact with eyes.

2. Keep out of the reach of children.

3. *Do not take internally* without consulting your health care practitioner. (Refer to Chapter Seven for recent research into the limited internal use of tea tree oil.) This precaution does not include the use of toothpaste, mouthwash (without swallowing), or douche.

4. For use in sensitive areas such as around the eyes, mouth, or genitals, dilute tea tree oil with alcohol or a good grade of cold-pressed oil such as olive, apricot, almond, or avocado.

5. Dilute with cold-pressed oil before use on baby's skin.

6. Do a patch test before using oil on sensitive skin. Extremely sensitive skin may need dilutions of the pure oil. Dilutions of

1:250 are still bacteriostatic against pathogenic streptococci and staphylococci, typhous, pneumococcus, and gonococcus.

7.   It is best to avoid alcoholic beverages (other than a glass of wine with your meal) if using essential oils.[4]

8.   Pregnant women should take extra precaution.

Patch Test

Put a few drops of tea tree oil on a cotton swab and apply to the inside of the arm. If you have an adverse reaction, irritation will appear on the skin within a matter of minutes. If the patch test doesn't indicate any irritation or allergic reaction, you may use a few drops of tea tree oil directly on the problem area of the skin once or twice a day.

Storage

Always keep tea tree oil in amber-colored bottles and store in a cool dry place. The oil will stay potent and will not deteriorate from exposure to light, air, and heat. *Do not store in plastic containers.* Cap should be on tight to avoid oxidation and evaporation.

Do not store or use tea tree oil near homeopathic remedies, as it may contaminate your remedy.

Shelf life is generally two to three years if properly stored. There have been reports of tea tree oil retaining its efficacy after being stored for much longer periods of time; however, perhaps due to stricter guidelines from various government regulatory bodies, it is now recommended that the oil be stored for a maximum of three years.

Use of tea tree oil should not be viewed as a substitute for professional medical care. If a problem persists, consult a doctor.

---

[4]*Better Nutrition*, August 1996.

Mixing Guide[5]

Water-Soluble Concentrate

1. Mix 1 oz. (2 tablespoons) full-strength tea tree oil and 1/2 oz. (1 tablespoon) isopropyl rubbing alcohol; shake well. If oil floats to the surface, add more alcohol and shake again. *Label for external use only.*

2. Mix 1 oz. full-strength tea tree oil with equal amount 192-proof Everclear alcohol, *or* three tablespoons 151-proof rum, *or* 6 tablespoons 80-proof alcohol (preferably vodka). Shake well.

3. Mix 1 oz. full-strength tea tree oil with 2 oz. (4 tablespoons) vegetable glycerine. Add 1 oz. water and shake well. If oil rises to the top, add more glycerine and shake again.

Mixtures 2 and 3 should be clearly labeled as "water-soluble tea tree oil concentrate." Since isopropyl alcohol is toxic, mixture #1 must be clearly labeled *for external use only.*

Fifteen Percent Solution

To make a 15 percent solution, take any of the above water-soluble tea tree oil concentrates and add enough water, herbal tea, aloe vera gel, or any combination of these to make 6 oz. (3/4 cup) of solution.

This 15 percent solution can be applied externally, used on infants and pets, and, if made with glycerine or grain alcohol (or vodka), may be used to treat mouth and gum conditions. Do *not* use the concentrate containing isopropyl alcohol for any mouth or gum or other internal conditions.

The 15 percent solution is good for spraying kitchen and bathroom surfaces, in air ducts and air conditioning units, on telephone receivers, in shower stalls, or adding to laundry water.

---

[5] Puotinen, C.J. *Nature's Antiseptics: Tea Tree Oil and Grapefruit Seed Extract.* New Canaan, CT; Keats Publishing, Inc., 1997.

Twenty Percent Oil Solution

To dilute tea tree oil in a carrier oil such as olive oil, add 1 oz. full-strength tea tree oil to 4 ozs. (1/2 cup) or more of the carrier oil. One ounce of tea tree oil in 4 ozs. carrier oil produces a 20 percent concentration of tea tree oil. This concentration is effective in treating a fungus condition such as athlete's foot.

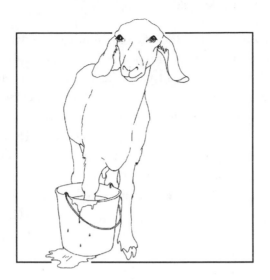

Chapter Four

Tea Tree Oil for Animals

"I've had milk goats for many years and I love them. They are hardy animals but things can go wrong. My favorite goat somehow got a bone infection in one leg. The vet said it's very hard to cure. We tried all the shots and pills he gave us to no avail. I tried another vet and used all the medication he gave us. No luck. Gangrene set in and we were talking about shooting her. Then a friend told me about Melaleuca—tea tree oil. I was ready to try anything! I put a few drops in a bucket of warm water and soaked her leg in it twice a day. After one week I saw improvement. After two weeks her leg was normal and hair was growing back. People couldn't believe the way she healed up. The next winter she started limping on that leg again and the hair started coming off. I soaked it in tea tree oil for a few days and she was fine." [6]

---

[6]*Countryside and Small Stock Journal*, Vol. 77, No. 5, September/October, 1993.

While living in Santa Barbara, California, I discovered that dogs and cats suffer immeasurably from allergies that create the "Santa Barbara itch." I witnessed my 14-year-old cat, Pepper, practically going crazy, scratching constantly. Out came the tea tree oil. I would smooth a few drops, diluted with water, onto her skin, and could practically hear her "meow" with relief. Today my cats Luna and Simba receive a pet spray containing tea tree before a brushing. Naturally, the oil is diluted to an amount that is good for them.

Tea tree oil is also an excellent flea repellent. You won't eliminate all the pesky critters; however, spraying the carpet with a tea tree oil mixture will help to control the fleas. It is a good idea to take pets outside before you wash them with tea tree shampoo so the fleas can jump off there rather than in the house. This goes for brushing their coats with the tea tree oil as well. Bathing your pet once a week helps to curb skin irritations.

Several years ago I received a call from Mark Blumenthal, who edits a publication called *HerbalGram* at the American Botanical Council in Austin, Texas and contributes many articles to various health food magazines and professional journals in the United States. He asked if I could give him some oil so he could treat a cat that had appeared at his door. The cat was wearing a flea collar that had gotten caught up under her leg and rubbed the skin raw, creating a large opening. Mark removed the collar and doused the area with a generous amount of tea tree oil. He used the oil for about two weeks and also used comfrey lanolin ointment and fresh aloe vera gel. He reported that the wound healed and left no scar. The cat adopted Mark and is still the office mascot at ABC more than ten years later.

Some time ago, a cat clinic reported that several cats had developed ringworm, with symptoms of hair loss, depression and nausea. The medicine normally prescribed could eat away their bone marrow, and to use it, the cats would have to be shaved, given a sulfur bath, and have their blood tested. Talk about trauma! The clinic made a formula of tea tree oil mixed with olive oil. Black walnut and cajuput oil were also used in the treatment. The cats responded well and an immediate improvement was noted, without resorting to the 'normal' treatment!

Tea Tree Oil for Cats and Dogs

The information in the remainder of this chapter is provided by Chey-anne West of **A Natural Path**, who has many years' experience treating animals with herbal and homeopathic remedies, using tea tree oil extensively in her work. A Natural Path is listed in the Resource Guide at the back of this book. Cheyanne's book on tea tree oil treatments for animals is also published by Kali Press.

Skin Conditions

Tea tree oil is very helpful in all kinds of skin conditions. When treating cats it is advised that you dilute tea tree oil in a mixture of water or oil, as their skin is more sensitive than a dog's.

Problem	Application
Bites, Cuts, Stings, Rashes, Vaccinations	place tea tree oil on a cotton ball and dab directly on area twice daily. For cats, dilute with olive or other cold-pressed oil.
Dermatitis	bathe animal thoroughly; remove hair around affected area and scrub with mild soap and water. Rub tea tree oil directly into the affected area twice daily until condition improves. Put animal into dry, clean cage or pet carrier; keep isolated to monitor condition and prevent contagious conditions from spreading.
Sunburn	keep area moist; mix equal parts tea tree and vitamin E oil. Apply in the evenings, keep animal out of the sun.
Warts	dab tea tree oil directly onto itching or bleeding warts to help soothe the pain and dry the area. It may take a few weeks of daily application to clear up the warts.

Lice, Mange, and Ringworm

Lice, mange, and ringworm usually affect unhealthy animals whose immune systems are weakened. All three conditions are contagious to humans as well as animals; isolate the animal during treatment.

Lice infestation is most common in the winter months. Dogs and cats that are around farm animals are most at risk. Mange is more common in dogs; rare in cats. Ringworm is more common in cats.

Problem	Application
Lice	bathe animal with mild soap and water; clip excess hair or shave area. Mix one tablespoon tea tree oil in one cup water; put mixture in spray bottle and spray affected areas to saturate. Leave solution on for ten minutes. Dry with paper towel and dispose. Use a cotton ball saturated with tea tree oil on stubborn areas. Repeat treatment daily for at least one week or until signs of lice are gone.
Mange	see directions for lice. Condition can be stubborn; consult your veterinarian for further suggestions. Keep animal isolated during treatment and disinfect kennel or carrier frequently.
Ringworm	clip hair away from affected area, scrub with mild soap and water. Apply tea tree oil or mixture directly onto area with cotton ball or swab. Treat twice daily for at least one week. Ringworm can be difficult to clear up, so stay with it. Confine animal in a kennel or carrier until ringworm is gone. Disinfect scissors, grooming tools, and treatment area as well as the kennel or carrier .

Ticks and Fleas

Fleas can cause a lot of problems. Dogs may chew raw spots on their skin; cats and dogs can become infected with tape and/or roundworms.

Problem	Application
Fleas	bathe animal with mild soap and water, clip hair from "hot spots." Mix one tablespoon tea tree oil into one cup water, put into spray bottle and spray animal down well; allow to stand for a few minutes, then saturate a cotton ball with tea tree oil and dab onto raw areas. Add a few drops of tea tree oil to pet shampoo for regular bathing. Shampoo and treat animal outdoors, so fleas won't jump off in your house.
Ticks	use an eyedropper to drop tea tree oil onto the tick and wait a minute or two. Then, grab the tick with tweezers and pull steadily for 5-10 seconds then twist and pull. This should pull out the head, too. To cut down on potential swelling and infection, drop another drop of tea tree oil onto the site and rub.

Abscesses and Puncture Wounds

Abscesses are more common in cats, and are usually the result of a fight. Abscesses and puncture wounds in dogs are typically caused by burrs or foxtails that get trapped in the hair and work their way into the skin.

Puncture wounds are usually quite narrow and deep, and the skin may rapidly heal over the surface, trapping bacteria and foreign matter in the wound. Abscesses will usually drain; if the area drains but does not heal, it may indicate foreign matter in the wound.

Always consider the severity of the wound; stitches may be required, or other treatment considered.

Abscesses and Puncture Wounds

Problem	Application
Abscesses and Puncture Wounds	clean area with warm water and mild soap. Put 1-2 drops tea tree oil directly onto site to cleanse wound and dissolve pus. If abscess is draining, keep area clean and continue putting tea tree oil twice daily until the site is clear of redness and a healthy scab has formed. For mouth ulcers or hard-to-reach areas, place a mixture of tea tree oil in a spray bottle and spray the area. Do not store the oil in plastic for more than a few days.

Liniment and Insect Repellent

Tea tree oil can be rubbed into a sore muscle or sprain to soothe and aid in circulation. Helpful for arthritis and other diseases of the joints and muscles. It is also a natural insect repellent. It can repel fleas, ticks, and some parasites as well.

Problem	Application
Sore Muscles, Sprains, Arthritis, Joint and Muscle Disorders	put a few drops of tea tree oil in your hand, along with massage or other oil. Rub into the affected area. If using a magnetic wrap, massage the area with oil mixture then wrap with clear plastic wrap before applying the magnetic wrap (follow directions for magnetic wrap). You may also use tea tree oil in conjunction with a heating pad; however, keep the pad on low to prevent burning the skin.
Repellent for Fleas, Ticks, Parasites	mix one teaspoon of tea tree oil in one cup water, put into a spray bottle, and before they go outside, spray your dog or cat to repel insects. This mixture may also be used to spray pet carriers or bedding to help keep the area free of pests.

Dental Problems

Tea tree oil relieves inflammation and abscesses in the mouth, and helps prevent infection. Both dogs and cats suffer from periodontal disease caused by a buildup of calcium salts, food, hair, and bacteria on the teeth. Symptoms include gum inflammation, swelling and bleeding, foul breath, and excessive salivation.

Problem	Application
Gum Disease, Foul Breath, Excessive Salivation	mix five drops tea tree oil into 1/4 cup water. Put mixture into squirt or spray bottle and spray area several times a day. You may also dip a toothbrush into this mixture and brush the teeth once a week to help keep bacteria down. Tea tree oil in the above solution will help heal and prevent infection when a tooth is decayed or removed.

Tea Tree Oil for Horses

For information about tea tree oil therapies for horses, please consult Cheyanne West's book: *Tea Tree Oil for Animals*, Kali Press, 1998.

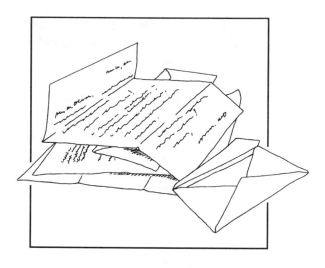

Chapter Five
Testimonials

*R*eports from Australian Practitioners[7]

re: Mouthwash —"I advise 5 drops to 4 ounces of water which I consider quite strong enough for cleansing and germicidal results."

re: Colitis —"Colitis with hemorrhage cured in two weeks. Bowel washed out frequently with a 1% solution and 5 drops of the pure oil 3 times a day taken internally."

re: Periostitis —"Suppurating bruise of shin which appeared to be progressing to a condition of periostitis, checked in 24 hours using solution diluted 1-40 as a compress. Condition cured in one week by continuing this treatment."

---

[7]Information provided by Thursday Plantation, Inc., Santa Barbara, California.

re: Halitosis —"In several cases of halitosis, especially after extraction, 5% or 1-20 dilution sprayed around the mouth gave almost instant relief within a few minutes."

re: Cuts, Bruises —"For superficial cuts, bruises and small contusions, the oil is painted on 100% and left to dry. A scab forms and healing under the scab almost invariably takes place within a few days.

re: Vaginal Cleansing —"I find in the saponified form that it is a very pleasant and efficient preparation for using in douches and for cleaning up discharges from the cervix uteri."

re: Colds —"Personally free from colds during the year, previously unknown. Personal friends relieved and cured of head and chest flu by inhaling (1) from a teaspoon of the pure oil in a pint of boiling water; (2) inserting a little of the pure oil in the nostril frequently."

re: Cleansing Wounds —A senior surgeon in a Sydney hospital had the following observations: "The results obtained in a variety of conditions when it [tea tree oil] was first tried were most encouraging, a striking feature being that it dissolved pus and left the surface of infected wounds clean so that its germicidal action became more effective and without any apparent damage to the tissues... Dirty wounds, such as are frequently seen as the result of street accidents... [the oil] will loosen and bring away the dirt which is usually ground in, and the tissues will remain fresh and retain their natural color."

Personal Testimonials

"Tea tree oil is good for infections. I also used it when I got some whiteheads and when I got a facial, the salon told me about tea tree oil being excellent for skin eruptions." MJ

"The inflamed cuts on my hand are gone...I have been in orthopedic treatment with aches—I put the stuff [tea tree oil] on and the aches went away." JG

"I'm a fan of tea tree oil...I mix it with a water miscible almond oil and use it to wash my face and apply to my scalp. It's cured my dandruff and itchy scalp." SF

"...my husband and I have been using the tea tree oil for the past two years for a variety of ailments... when we came down with sore throats, we gargled with a few drops in water and within a few days the sore throat was gone. I got a severe sunburn...the [tea tree] lotion not only took away the pain but I never did blister or peel." TL - El Toro, California

"After using tea tree oil for the past two to three years in my busy herbalist/naturopath practice...tea tree oil works really well with...impetigo, the herpes simplex blisters, and most types of ulcerous tissue...it replaces antibiotic powders. I carry your tea tree oil in the car and in my bag where I use it as a 'First Aid Kit in a Bottle.' " GS - herbal practitioner, Avalon, New South Wales

"I had chicken pox one year ago. I had it for two weeks, and the itching was incredible...I used calamine lotion...soaked a couple of times a day in an anti-itch oatmeal...As for essential oils, I put tea tree, ten drops; lavender, ten drops; and lemon, five drops— in two tablespoons of vegetable oil. I dabbed this mixture on the pox on my face a few times a day. My face healed faster than my body, and I have absolutely no scars on my face (my body has a few)." Anon.

"How grateful I am for your efforts and your book about tea tree oil...I have very sensitive skin and am tired of many other medicines and products that seem to hurt and dull my senses. I have used tea tree oil in taking sun, on my skin as a moisturizer...tonic on my hair...the oil helps soothe, heal and bring vitality to my skin, hair, and my sense of life. I work in a very toxic profession, as an artist for almost twenty years...the oil helps alleviate the harm the leads, zincs and powerful solvents have on my system...looking forward to having the aid of this unique natural gift for the rest of my life..." CG - Montecito, California

"My husband contracted a severe cement dust allergy...he was confined to a wheelchair...[the] skin of his feet and calves was so tender...caused bleeding and great pain...our doctor advised that it was most likely that amputation of both legs below the knee would be necessary...I purchased a bottle [of tea tree oil] and we rubbed it all over the affected area...Within two weeks the condition had cleared up totally and...there has been no recurrence whatsoever...Your tea tree oil is extraordinary." EM - Sydney, N.S.W.

"My clinic, 'The AIDS Alternative Health Project' is a donation-only clinic that serves 120 AIDS patients a week with 144 on a waiting list...Weekly visits to the clinic for treatment and a large home care routine, much of which includes your tea tree oil... Basically into every internal use–toothpaste, drops on tongue, in vaporizer, enemas, suppositories... While not a cure, I feel absolute success in candida control, skin infections, etc." AS - Chicago, IL

"Just a quick note to tell you how your great tea tree oil has helped my skin problem clear up." TA - San Marcus, California

"My son Rudie went to summer camp and came home just eaten up with mosquito bites all over his body. He was scratching them making matters worse. I applied your tea tree oil and in just 20 minutes the itching stopped and the next morning all was well." CC - Dallas, Texas

"Thank you, thank you, for the marvelous tea tree oil. I have been suffering from cold sores for years and they get quite bad at times to the point of leaving scar tissue on my face. My last bout with this problem was much better, thanks to your tea tree oil. In fact, as I felt it coming on, I started using the tea tree oil and it never developed into a sore." CD - Rockwall, Texas

"While at a health food trade show in Las Vegas three years ago, I learned about the amazing healing applications of tea tree oil. One area that particularly interested me was dental applications. At the age of 65, I was suffering from receding and bleeding gums. I purchased some oil and decided to put it to the test. I took the tea tree oil to my dentist and had a full checkup. I told him that I was going to rinse my mouth out twice a day with three drops of tea tree oil in a small cup of water, for three to five minutes.

"I must tell you that my dentist would get blood at almost every place on my gums. I also gave up flossing. The plan was to have a checkup every 30 days for a prolonged period of time. My first checkup after 30 days already began to show improvement. My dentist could draw blood in only six spots. In 60 days, there was no bleeding at all, even with the gums being deeply gouged. After 13 months of treatment, the gums stopped bleeding and the receding gums had returned to normal. The dentist said that the plaque and calculus had been reduced 75-80%. Tea tree oil saved my teeth. Aloha!" BMc - Oahu, Hawaii

"Thank you from the bottom, top and sides of my heart! Your tea tree oil is...wonderful...As a person with AIDS, I take massive doses of different drugs. These drugs dry my skin. The tea tree oil/cream helps to reverse this dryness and makes life a whole lot better..." JI - Washington, D.C.

"I have your books on tea tree oil .They are wonderful. I have found the oil to be most wonderful for so many things. I also would like to say that even though it took my dog a day or two to adjust to the scent of the tea tree oil, I have to date found nothing to compare to it for healing his small tumors and warts. It is truly a blessed oil..." MH

"I consider our discovery of...tea tree oil...to be one of the better things that happened to us in 1990. I've had arthritis for several years and find I get the greatest relief by applying tea tree to the affected joint (or area). A gargle solution of two or three drops of tea tree oil in a 1/4 cup of water certainly nips a threatening sore throat in the bud.

"I have always had a problem with plaque buildup on my teeth and have them cleaned every six months for that. After three months of adding a couple of drops of the oil to the toothpaste before brushing, I've experienced no plaque buildup and my teeth are definitely whiter.

"Cuts, burns, abrasions and insect bites heal so much more quickly with tea tree oil. I use the antiseptic lotion for vaginal cleanliness, as well as for extremely dry skin. My husband particularly likes tea tree soap and toothpaste." FB - Carlsbad, California

"Thanks for the information on tea tree oil. I am passing along the pertinent data to my vet...I am sure she will be interested, especially after seeing what it is doing with the viral growth on my horse's back. This is a viral growth called a sarcoid and it appears also to be diminishing with the use of the tea tree oil. The other bump which I eliminated doesn't have a name that I know of, but is like an infected ingrown hair. We continue to make these disappear on both of our horses' backs with tea tree oil..." JE - Scottsdale, Arizona

"To prevent dehydration of the skin in the airplane I use tea tree Antiseptic Lotion-I don't know what I would do without it." BD - Airline Captain of 29 years

"About four years ago we began to experience infestations of 'kissing bugs' or cone-nosed beetles in our house during May and June. The bugs always seemed to bite me at night while I was asleep. The next morning, I would have a huge lump at the location of the bite, and it would be itchy and painful. It generally took 2-3 days for the lump to go away. Nothing of the medications I used seemed to help, until I tried tea tree oil. When I first discovered a bite, I rubbed in some of the oil and kept doing so at frequent intervals. Relief of the itching was almost immediate, and within 6-8 hours of the first application of the oil, the swelling was drastically reduced. I definitely plan to keep my medicine cabinet stocked with tea tree oil." DB - Fountain Hills, AZ

A new suggestion received by a reader: "A sea sponge may be used instead of tampons for vaginal infections. Simply cut the sponge to fit inside the vagina and insert. When sponge is full, remove, rinse thoroughly with warm water, and reinsert. At the end of the cycle, the sponge has to dry out in the sun. *Failure to do this can create bacteria from the moisture.* The sponge can then be soaked in tea tree oil (a few drops) diluted with water to kill the bacteria if this does occur. The same sponge can be used for six months." NC - Radford, VA

"I went to our local health food store and found the incredible book Tea Tree Oil First Aid Handbook. I myself had a very difficult time looking tea tree oil up in my local library... to enlighten people about this marvelous source of nature's best... I can't help being excited about it. I use the products, thank you for a great book." VM

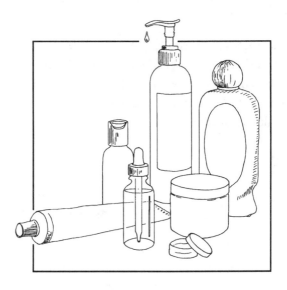

Chapter Six

Tea Tree Oil Products

$\mathcal{L}$ ooking Good the Healthy Way

Many French cosmetic manufacturers, and recently U.S. companies, are using tea tree essential oil in toiletry and cosmetic formulations that include lip balm, body lotion, moisturizer, deodorant, shower gels, toothpaste, mouthwashes, and dental floss. Tea tree's spicy aroma adds appeal when mixed into soaps, shampoos, lotions, and perfumes. Some of the more elegant New York City salons are using tea tree oil as a pre-manicure/pedicure soak. Tea tree oil contains antiseptic and anti-fungal properties to help combat bacteria, thus the salon soaks help to eliminate athlete's foot and nail fungus.

Tea tree skin cream helps to oxygenate skin cells while aiding in the repair of damaged skin caused by sun, acne, dry skin, fungus, and various other skin ailments. Skin takes on a youthful glow. In fact, the

U.S. government has approved the use of tea tree oil in cosmetic formulations. The oil contains very low levels of toxicity. Tea tree oil is non-irritating to almost all areas of the body and at times, depending on the application and treatment, will help dead tissue slough off to allow healthy skin to appear.

Face and Body Care

In this day and age, more people are becoming susceptible to viral conditions such as cold sores. Since cold sores usually appear on the face and around the mouth, the infected individual may become self-conscious about the outbreak. Often cold sores can be controlled by applying a few drops of pure tea tree oil onto the infected area at the onset. The oil will help to keep the cold sore from manifesting.

Dermatitis, dry skin, fungus, corns, and athlete's foot are just a few skin problems that we all face at one time or another. Generally, dry skin brushing and using a body lotion with tea tree oil added will help to repair and smooth the injured skin. Bathing in tea tree oil is therapeutic and soothing for tired muscles. Add ten drops of the oil to a warm tub and soak for twenty minutes. It is not necessary to use much oil; I once had a call from a woman who added an entire ounce to her tub, sat in hot water for one hour, and her skin turned bright red. Remember, a little goes a long way.

"For persistent or extensive infections by athlete's foot fungus, doctors often prescribe an oral antibiotic called griseofulvin. It is expensive, can be toxic, has to be taken for long periods of time, especially if the nails are affected, and often fails to eliminate the infection. Tea tree oil is cheap, safe and more effective, even for diseased nails."

Andrew Weil, M.D.
Natural Health, Natural Medicine

Tea tree oil has been known to penetrate to the cellular level. Try adding ten drops of pure oil to your favorite day or night cream to help moisturize and smooth skin.

After shaving or waxing, apply several drops of the oil to the newly waxed or shaved area. It helps to cut down redness or swelling. A lotion containing a few drops of tea tree oil will also work well. Ingrown hairs can be eliminated by massaging the oil into the skin. This method is effective for both men and women.

Nail Care

Within the last several years, there has been an increase in the occurrence of parionychia, a fungal infection which appears on fingernails and toenails, due to the popularity of acrylic and silk nail applications, or in some cases, harsh detergents. Many women have their nails redone every two weeks; sometimes when nails are applied, moisture may get trapped in the nail bed. If this happens, a lifting of the nail may occur within a week and a half. If left untreated, a fungus could develop. Three stages of nail fungus occur:

Stage 1: If moisture occurs and the nail begins to lift, and is left untreated, a light green stain will appear on the nail bed.

Stage 2: The nail bed will turn dark green.

Stage 3: The nail bed will eventually turn black. A light yellow tinge usually indicates a nail fungus as well.

There have been horror stories about women refusing to treat their nail fungus and asking their nail salon to cut back the infected nail and slap another nail on top. A good salon will refuse to do this due to the poor condition of the nail. Dramatic results have been achieved by applying tea tree oil on, around, and under the nail bed, rubbing in several drops twice a day. For mildew, use a good tea tree oil soap, or a mixture of a few drops of tea tree oil in liquid soap, massage onto the nail plate and wash off all residue. It is important to have nails free of any oil so that the new nail application will adhere properly. To remove nail stains, buff the nail with iodine and tea tree oil. The nail will dry to a milky white color. Buff off the milky white to remove all the stain from the nail.

Hair Care

Both sexes tease, color, mousse, blow-dry, and perm their hair. Not only do these treatments dry the hair, but the hair follicle itself can be blocked, creating further problems such as hair thinning and loss. A tea tree oil shampoo, or any natural shampoo with 2% tea tree oil (ten drops to an eight-ounce bottle), will help to unblock clogged hair follicles, moisturize the hair and keep the scalp free of bacteria and fungal problems.

Dry hair requires a gentle, non-detergent based product; a 2% solution of tea tree oil in a moisturizing shampoo will help to unblock sebaceous glands and encourage the flow of the body's own moisturizing oils, while clearing away unsightly dead skin cells.

For oily hair, a gentle tea tree oil moisturizing shampoo will help cleanse the scalp of bacterial and fungal irritations and help to disperse dead skin cells.

Tea tree oil mixed with other essential oils is especially good as a scalp treatment for relieving dandruff. Medical professionals list infection, poor diet, blood circulation and inadequate nerve stimulation as some of the causes of dandruff. A yeast that lives on the scalp, *Pityrosporum ovale,* and a fungus called *trichoplyton spp* also contribute to dandruff conditions. While there are many anti-fungal and bacterial soaps and shampoos on the market, tea tree oil offers a natural alternative. A recent study indicates that a pharmaceutical grade of tea tree oil in low concentrations helps to eliminate bacteria and fungus on the scalp, as well as Pityrosporum ovales. There have also been reports that by massaging the oil into the scalp, new hair growth is promoted.

Hair Treatments for Children

When my grandchildren were little, my daughter called and asked if she could use the tea tree oil as a treatment for cradle cap. I suggested that she take one part of pure oil and mix it with ten parts of another oil, such as almond oil. She could gently massage the oil into the baby's scalp and leave it on for a few minutes, then follow up with a tea tree shampoo. My daughter called back a few days later and reported that the cradle cap was gone!

It seems that at the beginning of every school year there is an outbreak of head lice among school children. The head lice, appearing as small greyish white specks, bite and puncture the scalp, causing pain and itching. The problem may persist due to the hatching of new eggs approximately every two weeks. Since head lice is contagious, it can be widespread. Head lice is often transmitted by combs, brushes, hats, bed linens, etc. I once spoke to a Dallas school nurse who voiced concern regarding the use of chemically-based shampoos—the standard treatment for children's head lice. She expressed a great deal of interest in being able to offer tea tree oil as a natural substitute.

The following treatment for removal of head lice is recommended: Add five to ten drops of pure tea tree oil to a shampoo and wash the child's hair, massaging this mixture thoroughly into the scalp. Do this every day until the eggs are removed. In between shampoos, a few drops of the oil can be massaged into the scalp. Do not rinse out. To help sterilize and prevent further lice infestation, brushes, combs, bedding, and towels may be soaked in a tea tree oil solution of 1/4 oz. of oil added to a tub of water. You may also spray a dilution of tea tree oil in the clothes hamper to help control infestation.

Dental Hygiene

Many Australian dentists use tea tree oil as a mouthwash and for sterilizing cavities before filling. Studies have shown that washing the mouth out twice a day with a few drops of tea tree oil will help to inhibit the growth of bacteria, and reports state that gum bleeding has been greatly reduced and plaque controlled.

Reports indicate that using tea tree oil in dental hygiene and in surgery show it to be an extremely effective antiseptic.

According to C.J. Puotinen in *Nature's Antiseptics,* holding a dilute solution of tea tree oil in your mouth for as long as possible before swishing and spitting it out will help with bleeding gums, inflammation, or infection in the mouth.

Tea Tree Oil in Aromatherapy

Aromatherapy is the use of essential oils, which may produce extraordinary individual changes on a physical, emotional, mental, or spiritual level.

An essential oil is the highly concentrated essence of a plant material, often extracted by a steam distillation process. Essential oils can be mixed with vegetable oils or alcohol, blended into massage lotions, bath oils, cosmetics, and perfume, used with facial masks, compresses, and in saunas and diffusers. The oils help to balance, rejuvenate, and stimulate the body and skin. Many body care products such as shampoos and creams are now being formulated with at least a 1% tea tree oil solution. Because some consumers have difficulty with the pungent scent of tea tree oil, fragrances such as jasmine and rose may be added in small concentrations (0.3 to 0.5%).

Each essential oil contains its own quality. The French gathered clinical data on tea tree oil in the mid-1980's (refer to Chapter Seven: Practitioners' Guide). Robert Tisserand, an English aromatherapist, has discussed tea tree oil in his books, *Aromatherapy for Everyone* and *The Art of Aromatherapy*. In the International Journal of Aromatherapy, February 1988, Mr. Tisserand called tea tree oil one of the most exciting essential oils to emerge in recent years.

Tea tree oil has long been recognized as a powerful antiseptic and fungicide, shown to be twelve to thirteen times stronger than carbolic acid, at one time the world's number-one antiseptic. Thus, tea tree is excellent as a first aid oil to help alleviate fungus on finger and toenails and on the skin. As a massage it can be blended with other oils to refresh the skin and to help keep the skin clean and healthy. As a bath soak, ten drops in a tub will help ease sore and injured muscles and joints, as well as infections of the skin. I have applied several drops in the humidifier to keep the air in my home clean. I put a few drops of tea tree oil into a diffuser I purchased several years ago from an essential oil company, and the aroma is like sitting in a grove of tea trees in the Australian bush! My daughter has used a few drops in a vaporizer which gives tremendous relief to the children when they come down with the sniffles.

Tea tree oil definitely can be added to the list of other fine essential oils as a great contribution to aromatherapy. Remember to store the pure oil in amber glass bottles to protect from heat and light, and keep in a cool place. If you mix small amounts of tea tree oil into other lotions, plastic is suitable. Refer to Chapter Three for more tea tree oil applications.

Products Containing Tea Tree Oil

Soaps—tea tree oil soap has shown to be very effective for skin blemishes, irritations, and as a general antiseptic. Many people with sensitive skin have reported the soap to be effective as well as mild, causing no skin irritation. Using the soap on a daily basis is beneficial for acne, cuts, abrasions, foot conditions, fungal irritations, and rashes.

Shampoo—a tea tree shampoo helps to control dandruff, itchy scalp, ringworm, lice, and seborrhea (see Chapter Three). Using shampoo on a daily basis or alternating with other naturally-based shampoos is recommended.

Antiseptic Cream—a therapeutic cream containing at least 5% tea tree oil helps heal diaper rash, sunburns, cuts, mosquito bites, rashes, athletes foot, and a number of other skin irritations.

Douche—yeast infections and candida have become prevalent in today's society because of eating habits, stress, accumulation of antibiotic treatments, moist conditions, etc. (See Chapter Seven for the test by Dr. Paul Belaiche of France in 1985.) A pessary product can be used vaginally and in the anal passage for difficulties such as hemorrhoids. A 2% solution of tea tree oil in a cocoa butter base has been effective in inhibiting the growth of infection without disturbing the body's natural flora. Use should be under medical supervision.

A tea tree oil douche has also been used for infections. Eight to ten drops of oil in a pint of purified or distilled water and douching in between pessary applications seems to help in reducing irritation, discomfort, and infection.

Tea Tree Toothpaste—tea tree toothpaste may prove to be effective for gingivitis, halitosis, plaque control and pyorrhea, as well as in dental surgery (refer to Case Studies, Chapter Seven).

Tea Tree Mouthwash—tea tree mouthwash is used to help prevent and treat periodontal disease and other mouth conditions. Many Australian dentists use tea tree oil as a mouthwash and to sterilize cavities before filling. Studies have shown that washing the mouth out twice a day with a few drops of tea tree oil will help to inhibit the growth of bacteria, and reports state that gum bleeding has been greatly reduced and plaque controlled.

Tea Tree Oil Deodorant—many of the deodorant products out today contain aluminum and other ingredients that may or may not be beneficial. Here again is another area where tea tree oil can play a role as a healthier alternative. Because tea tree oil is 10-13 times stronger than carbolic acid (once considered the number one antiseptic in the world), a tea tree oil deodorant may help to minimize risk of bacteria buildup and razor burns as well.

Anti-Itch Pet Shampoos—skin allergies in animals lead to itching and chaffing of the skin, and many animals have scratched themselves raw. A pet shampoo containing tea tree oil, if used once or twice a week, can help heal the irritation, stop the itching, promote a healthy coat, and control fleas. Be sure to leave the pet shampoo on for three to five minutes before you rinse. This product is beneficial for dogs, cats and horses. This is an excellent alternative to the toxic "dips" done in many veterinary offices.

For more information on tea tree products for animals, refer to Chapter Four, "Tea Tree Oil for Animals."

The Marketplace

Several years ago, the Australian division of the Colgate-Palmolive Company offered a product called "Protex" germicidal soap. The main ingredient was tea tree oil. Their slogan was "Did you Protex yourself this morning?" Colgate's U.S. parent company wanted to produce the soap for mass market, but there simply was not enough oil available at the time. Eventually the Australian Colgate company stopped producing the germicidal soap in favor of scented soap.

Several Australian and American companies are now producing an entire line of tea tree products and are adding the oil to their existing or new formulations. Sun screens, mouthwash, lozenges, massage oils, creams and lotions are now appearing on the shelves in health food and body-care stores throughout the United States. One company boasts the production of over sixty products made with tea tree oil, which include biodegradable household cleaning items.

Tea tree oil is also being used by chiropractors for the relief of muscle tightness as well as for skin irritations. Another tea tree product that proves useful for professionals as well as for individuals is a salve for sore muscles. Tea tree oil products have been used in Australia by naturopaths for some time for the treatment of thrush. In Switzerland the oil is used to control infections in hospitals; an Australian industrial company uses it in a product to help sterilize air-conditioning and venting systems in public buildings to aid in the control of Legionnaire's Disease.

Meanwhile, tea tree oil is becoming more visible in the mass marketplace. Hair salon products include tea tree oil shampoos. Mail order catalogs are beginning to include tea tree oil and products in their lines. With the increased awareness of herbal products in mainstream consciousness, the immediate future holds exciting possibilities for tea tree oil in many different marketplaces.

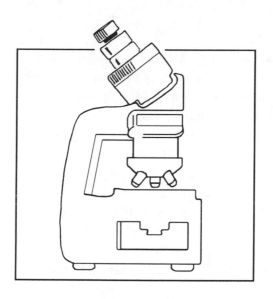

Chapter Seven

Practitioners' Guide

*C*ase Studies

Pena Study: Yeast Infections

In the late 1950's and the early 1960's, Dr. Eduardo F. Pena, M.D. investigated Melaleuca alternifolia oil for effectiveness in eradicating both trichomonal vaginitis and candida.[8] A further purpose of this study was to observe any possible irritation or side effects and to determine the proper strength of the oil for safety and efficacy. The solution consisted of an emulsified 40% solution of Australian Melaleuca alternifolia oil with 13% isopropyl alcohol. This special emulsion results in the solution being miscible (able to mix) with water in all proportions, giving a milky appearance when diluted.

---

[8] *Obstetrics and Gynecology*, June 1962.

The study was conducted on 130 women suffering from four types of vaginal infections: 96 cases of trichomonal vaginitis, several cases of thrush and cervicitis, and a control group of 50 women who were treated with anti-trichoma suppositories. Out of 130 patients, all treatment was successful and the tea tree oil treatments had similar results to the control group. In the 96 cases of trichomonal vaginitis, clinical cures were obtained by inserting a tampon saturated with a 1% solution of Melaleuca alternifolia oil which was then removed after 24 hours. Daily vaginal douches of 1% solution in one quart of water were also recommended. The number of office treatments necessary to achieve a clinical cure averaged 6, while the total number of douches per patient averaged 42. Patients commented about the pine odor and soothing, cooling effect of the tea tree oil. It was also apparent that at no time did the patient experience irritation or burning.

The clinical study indicated that tea tree oil is a penetrating germicide and fungicide with the additional characteristics of dissolving pus and debris.

H.M. Feinblatt, 1960

Melaleuca alternifolia oils were applied at full strength to boils two or three times daily, with outstanding success. Rapid healing was reported, without scarring. It was believed that the improvement in the condition of the boils was caused by the high germicidal effect of the oil against *Staphylococcus aureus* in the presence of pus. There were no toxic effects as a result of this treatment.[9]

M. Walker, Foot Problems, April, 1972

In a 1972 study[10] done on various foot problems, i.e.: athlete's foot, fungal infections, under-toenail corns, and callouses, Dr. Walker used tea tree oil in three different formulas: first as a pure oil; second, 40% oil with 13% isopropyl alcohol (which allows the oil to be water miscible, giving it another name, Melasol) and third, 8% oil with lanolin

---

[9]*Journal of the National Medical Association*, 1960. 52(1):32-34
[10]*Current Podiatry*, April 1972.

and chlorophyll. Sixty patients were involved in the study. Forty were put on Melasol, 20 applied the ointment and 8 used the pure oil. Treatments varied from three weeks to four years. Out of 68 patients, 58 found relief from their foot problems over a period of six years. At least four different fungal conditions are affiliated with athlete's foot, all of which responded well using tea tree oil.

Belaiche, First Study: Thrush (Candida albicans) September, 1985

Dr. Paul Belaiche, Chief of Phytotherapy Department at the Faculty of Medicine, University of Paris, has worked on several studies involving tea tree oil. One study was conducted on patients with thrush, a vaginal infection of *Candida albicans*.[11] Although there are normally low levels of candida found in the vagina, the growth is kept under control

> *"The essential oil of Melaleuca has entered the team of major essential oils and emerges as an antiseptic and antifungal weapon of the first order in phyto-aromatherapy."*
>
> Dr. Paul Belaiche

by certain bacteria. It is when an increasing amount of antibiotic treatment is used that the healthy bacteria cease to flourish and the candida proliferates. Some indications of infection are itching, white discharge and pain.

Dr. Belaiche's study focused on 28 patients using a tea tree oil suppository inserted into the vagina every evening. One week later, one patient discontinued treatment due to vaginal burning. Thirty days later, upon examination 21 out of 28 patients showed a complete recovery. The remaining seven were clinically, but not biologically, cured. Dr. Belaiche felt tea tree oil to be very effective, less irritating than other essential oils, and easily tolerated by vaginal membranes.

Belaiche: Second Study, Chronic Cystitis

Twenty-six female patients, average age of 39, were given a capsule of tea tree oil once a day over a three-month period. Because this was a

---

[11]*Phytotherapie*, Vol. 15, 1985.

"From this first clinical approach, it is apparent that the essential oil of Melaleuca alternifolia is effectively efficient for the treatment of chronic colibacilli cystitis."

Dr. Paul Belaiche

double-blind study, there were two lots of 13 patients each. Lot A was given 24 mgs. of Melaleuca alternifolia daily—three doses of 8 mgs. before main meals. Lot B received a placebo. After six months, Lot B showed no improvement, while in Lot A, 7 (out of 13) were cured.[12]

Bacterial Vaginosis

A patient having been diagnosed with bacterial vaginosis refused a pharmaceutical drug (metronidazole) and instead used tea tree oil pessaries which contained 200 mg. of tea tree oil. The treatment lasted five days and a one-month follow-up showed the condition cleared. Tea tree oil may be a safe, non-toxic alternative to standard antibiotic therapy.[13]

Acne Study Done by Lederle Laboratories and Royal Prince Alfred Hospital, Fall 1990

Benzoyl Peroxide Versus Tea Tree Oil

An acne study was completed in the fall of 1990 comparing 5% benzoyl peroxide water-based lotion with a gel containing 5% tea tree oil.[14] Five of the 124 patients that participated did not complete the study because they had been on antibiotics for treatment of other illnesses. Sixty-one people were in the benzoyl group and 58 in the tea tree group. No topical acne treatment was used two weeks prior to the trial study.

Due to the difference in color and aroma between the two acne treatments, the three-month study was conducted as a single blind study; the investigator being "blind." Also, none of the patients were aware of which treatment they were receiving.

[12]*Phytotherapy*, September 1985. No. 115, pp. 9-11
[13]*Lancet*, December 8, 1989.
[14]*Medical Journal of Australia*, Vol. 153, No. 8

The study showed a 5% tea tree oil gel was effective as a topical acne treatment; however, due to the slower onset of action, it was less effective than the benzoyl lotion. Benzoyl's action may be due to established properties as a keratolytic agent, which tea tree oil probably does not have.

Although the tea tree solution was slower acting, after one month's time, 79% of the benzoyl group experienced greater dryness, pruritus, stinging, burning, and redness, versus 44% in the tea tree group. Tea tree oil was also better tolerated by facial skin.

Since the tea tree oil gel was administered at only 5% solution, another study may be done using higher concentrations of the oil. According to anecdotal reports, acne has been treated successfully in the past using 100% tea tree oil.

This acne study was the first to compare tea tree oil to a common pharmaceutical preparation in a clinically controlled trial. Also, it is important to note that a major pharmaceutical company conducted the test.

1991 Tea Tree Oil Study.
Dr. Alvin Shemash, Family Practitioner

Tea tree oil was tested on 50 patients with skin problems, chosen at random.[15] The purpose was to test and confirm the efficacy and safety of high quality tea tree oil. Several varieties of the oil were used including the pure oil (100%); lozenges with 1% oil and some of the ground leaf; and a 5% cream).

The 50 patients tested consisted of 18 men, 30 women and 2 children, ages ranging from 4 to 93. The treatment lasted from one to four weeks depending on the severity of the condition to be treated. One patient dropped out of the study and a second discontinued due to a mild erythematous skin sensitivity to the 100% oil. This was the only side-effect reported.

---

[15] In cooperation with William Mayo, Ph.D., President, American Society for Environmental Education.

The results of using the tea tree oil were striking. All patients but one were cured or showed remarkable improvement of the conditions treated. In the single case of eczema resistant to the oil, the pruritus decreased. The doctor also noted that tea tree oil is a natural, less costly, effective alternative to drugs, with fewer side effects.

The table below summarizes the conditions that were treated:

Condition	No. of Patients	Product Used
Mild facial & back acne	8	Cream
Monilia of throat/mouth	13	Lozenges
Monilial rashes of skin	6	Cream
Non-specific dermatitis, eczema	4	Oil/Cream
Infected pustules	1	Oil
Oral canker sores	3	Oil
Herpes simplex–face & lips	6	Oil
Fungus of fingernails, tinea cruris, pedis & barbae	7	Oil/Cream
Total Patients	48	

Podiatry Training Clinic, Sydney, Australia

Geriatric Test

A study completed by Dr. Jill Fogarty at Royal North Shore Hospital in Sydney used hand and body lotion containing a 5% solution of tea tree oil. The purpose of the study was to compare the skin on the legs of diabetic and geriatric patients. The 70 people in the study suffered from dry skin and/or debilitating diseases such as diabetes.

The patients were asked to use the cream for a period of 25-26 days, on one leg only. A marked difference was noticed on the leg that received the tea tree oil cream. Dry skin became much softer, cracks healed and disappeared. Tea tree oil's potential as a bactericide and skin emollient was noted. This study is important due to the ages of the people whose thin, fragile skin may be easily damaged and take longer to heal.

Treatment of Nail Fungus: A Comparison of Two Topical Preparations

D.S. Buck, D.M. Nidorf, and J.G. Addino[16]

Standard treatments for fungal infection of the nails *(onychomycosis)* include debridement (removal of foreign matter and dead or damaged tissue), topical medication, and systemic therapies. This study assesses the efficacy and tolerability of topical applications of 1% clotrimazole solution compared with that of 100% Melaleuca alternifolia (tea tree) oil for the treatment of toenail onychomycosis.

In a six-month double-blind, multicenter, randomized controlled trial of 117 patients with distal subungual onychomycosis, participants received twice-daily applications of either 1% clotrimazole (CL) solution (topical antifungal drug), or 100% tea tree (TTO) oil. Debridement and clinical assessment were performed at 0, 1, 3, and 6 months; cultures obtained at 0 and 6 months. After 6 months, the two groups were comparable based on culture cure (CL=11%, TTO=18%). Three months later, approximately half of each group reported continued improvement or resolution.

It was concluded that, while all current therapies have high recurrence rates, the use of a topical preparation in conjunction with debridement is an appropriate initial treatment. Topical therapy, including the above two preparations, provides improvement in nail appearance and symptoms, while oral therapy has the disadvantage of high cost and potentially serious adverse effects.

This study reinforces the need to use a potent (in this case 100%) concentration of tea tree oil to produce better short-term and long-term efficacy. In children and those with skin sensitivity, a 70% solution may be better tolerated.

---

[16]*Journal of Family Practice*, 1994. Jun; 38(6):601-5.

Animal Studies: St. Ives Veterinary Clinic, Australia; Spring 1988

For the previous sixteen to eighteen months, treatment trials were pre-scribed using a tea tree oil shampoo for a variety of skin ailments, most noticeably of an allergic and/or pruritic nature. Annabelle Olsson, the Superintendent, reported that the tea tree oil shampoo was a success as an "anti-itch" treatment and that in 80% of the cases, pruritus was controlled or diminished. She also noted that regular bathing with the shampoo helped decrease the flea population, as well as improve the condition of the animals' coats.

The following case histories summarize the animal testing reported by Ms. Olsson:

Labrador Retriever, 6-year-old spayed female
  History: eczema and fleas.
  Therapy: tea tree oil shampoo once a week. Within two weeks, coat condition improved. Flea rinse only required every two weeks.
Cat, 10-year-old neutered male
  History: chronic dermatitis and "hot spots" behind ears.
  Therapy: tea tree oil shampoo every 1-2 weeks. Also, pure tea tree oil directly on the coat. The dermatitis was reduced dramatically.
Australian Cattle Dog, 4-year-old spayed female.
  History: flea allergy and trauma.
  Therapy: tea tree oil shampoo weekly. For the last six months, fleas are minimal.
Pekingese, 14-year-old male
  History: fungal lesions on neck and chest.
  Therapy: tea tree oil shampoo daily. Tea tree oil applied after bath. Within five days, improvement dramatic. In three weeks, lesions completely gone.
Cocker Spaniel/Poodle. 8-year-old male
  History: chronic flea allergy dermatitis. Animal attacking its tail.

Therapy: iodine scrub, tea tree oil shampoo weekly. Reduced problem within two weeks.

Golden Retriever, 9-year-old spayed female

History: nervous dog with skin allergies. Fleas severe in summer.

Therapy: tea tree oil shampoo twice a week. Owner discontinued treatment against veterinarian's advice.

Labrador/Setter, 8-year-old male

History: chronic pruritus and hair loss on rump, flanks, thighs and abdomen.

Therapy: tea tree oil shampoo weekly. Within three weeks, hair began to regrow. Six months later, dog has healthy coat and receives regular tea tree oil shampoos.

Cat, 14-year-old neutered male

History: flea allergy dermatitis.

Therapy: tea tree oil shampoo 1-2 times a week. Hair began to regrow within two weeks.

It must be noted that in all cases the animals had been treated with drugs such as meoestral or prednisolone during their previous treatments. In some cases, steroids were continued for only a short period of time. Preventative maintenance including healthy diets and clean environment were important steps in the animals' recoveries.

Clinical Research Data

Source: Carson, C.F., B.D. Cookson, H.D. Farrelly, and T.V. Riley. "Susceptibility of methicillin-resistant *Staphylococcus aureus* to the essential oil of Melaleuca alternifolia." *Journal of Antimicrobial Chemotherapy*, 1995. 35:421-424

Hospital patients are susceptible to contact with infectious bacteria that can be easily transmitted through hospital staff members. One such common bacteria is *Staphylococcus aureus*. The bacteria was tested for antibiotic resistance. Tea tree oil dilutions of 0.2% - 2.0% were added to the cultures of the bacteria, and growth measured. The effective tea tree dosage to inhibit the bacteria was 0.25%; 0.5% killed the bacteria. There were few side effects from skin irritation. These in-vitro results suggest tea tree oil may be useful in the treatment of MRSA carriage.

Source: Carson C.F. et al. "Susceptibility of Propionibacterium acnes to the essential oil of Melaleuca alternifolia." Letter in *Applied Microbiology*, 1994. 19(1):24-25.

Propionibacterium Acnes: in vitro the bacteria associated with the acne was susceptible to tea tree oil; however, skin products were not as effective as benzoyl peroxide. Minimum inhibitory concentrations (mic) were difficult to establish for an essential oil causing turbidity when introduced into the growth medium; instead researchers were limited to analyzing minimum bactericidal concentrations (mbc's).

Source: Carson, C.F., T.V. Riley. "Antimicrobial activity of the major components of the essential oil of Melaleuca alternifolia." *Journal of Applied Bacteriology*, 1995b. 78(3): 264-269.

The antimicrobial activity of eight components of tea tree oil was evaluated using disc diffusion and broth microdilution methods. Attempts were also made to overcome problems encountered with testing compounds which have limited solubility in aqueous media. The disc diffusion method was used to determine the susceptibility of a range of micro-organisms to 1,8-cineole, 1-terpinen-4-ol, rho-cymene, linalool, alpha-terpinene, gamma-terpinene, alpha-terpineol, and terpinolene. The disc diffusion method lacked reproducibility, but was considered useful to screen for antimicrobial activity.

Terpinen-4-ol was active against all the test organisms; linalool and alpha-terpineol were active against all organisms except *Pseudomonas aeruginosa*; rho-cymene showed no antimicrobial activity. Minimum inhibitory and minimum cidal concentrations of each component against *Candida albicans*, *Escherichia coli* and *Staphylococcus aureus* were determined using a broth microdilution method. Modifications to this method overcame solubility and turbidity problems and allowed the antimicrobial activity of each of the components to be quantified reproducible. There was reasonable agreement between minimum inhibitory concentrations and zones of inhibition. These results may have significant implications for the future development of tea tree oil as an antimicrobial agent.

Source: Smith, Martha D., Patricia L. Navilliat. "A new protocol for antimicrobial testing of oils." *Journal of Microbiological Methods* 28 (1997) 21-24.

This paper is concerned with bactericidal testing of oil distilled from the tea tree *(Melaleuca alternifolia* and *M. linariifolia)* for FDA recognition of tea tree oil as a safe and effective topical ingredient. It would be the first natural topical antiseptic so recognized. The difficulty in testing tea tree oil is that the pure oil is not water soluble, and floats to the top of the bacterial medium. The FDA's proposed method for testing has been to use water-soluble and/or miscible products together with a chemical neutralizer.

In this test, a protocol was established to test the oil in a non-water-soluble form, using a non-toxic solvent. Tea tree oil demonstrated the FDA required bactericidal 3 $\log_{10}$ kill against *Pseudomonas aeruginosa, Staphylococcus aureus*, and *Escherichia coli*. These three organisms have been selected by the FDA because of their prevalence and life-threatening potential. The authors have petitioned the FDA to include this new protocol in proposed 21 CFR 333.71 (d) ii, "Bactericidal Assay Procedures" in the testing monograph for First Aid Antiseptic Drug Products.

Source: Bishop, C.D. "Antiviral activity of the essential oil of Melaleuca alternifolia (Maiden and Betche) Cheel (Tea tree) against tobacco mosaic virus." *Journal of Essential Oil Research,* 1995. 7:
641-644.
  In this antiviral study, tea tree oil was applied to *Nicotinia
glutinosa* plants which were then inoculated with tobacco mosaic virus at 100, 200 and 500 ppm. The tea tree oil reduced the
number of virus-induced lesions on the plants. It is unknown
whether the high amount of terpinen-4-ol in tea tree oil attrib-
uted to the antiviral effect, or if other essential oils would have
the ability to interact with the virus.

Source: *Tea Tree Oil News;* the Main Camp Tea Tree Oil Group Newsletter; November/December 1996 - January 1997. A collaborative study
between the Australian Tea Tree Oil Research Institute (ATTORI) and
the University of Western Sydney (UWS).
  Legionnaire's disease (or legionellosis), a form of pneumonia
caused by the *Legionella pneumophila* bacteria, is commonly
spread through inhalation of small droplets of water, usually
from poorly designed and/or maintained air-conditioning systems. Though this pneumonia is normally treated with antibiotics, it has proven it can be fatal, particularly among the elderly.
In-vitro trials conducted as part of the above collaborative study
indicate that in concentrations as low as 0.1%, Main Camp pharmaceutical grade tea tree oil kills this bacteria. ATTORI hopes
to further this work with pilot scale studies on airborne delivery
systems.

Source: Williams, Dr. Lyall; Vicki Home. School of Chemistry,
Macquarie University, Sydney, NSW, Australia. "A comparative study
of some essential oils for potential use in topical applications for the
treatment of the yeast *Candida albicans.*"[17]
  While the activity of synthetic antifungal drugs may be stronger

---

than tea tree oil against Candida albicans, many vaginal infections are a result of multiple infections involving bacteria and yeasts. In these circumstances, tea tree oil with a broad spectrum of antimicrobial activity against both yeast and other bacteria, coupled with additional properties of stability and non-irritancy, is ideal for incorporation into formulations for vaginal conditions. For Candida albicans, tea tree oil levels of 3-5% are effective.

Source: Tisserand, Robert. *The International Journal of Aromatherapy*, February 1988. Referenced in article by Frank Murray, "Vitamins/Supplements," *Better Nutrition for Today's Living*, Vol. 56, No. 4, April 1994.

Tisserand states that tea tree oil has passed the Kelsey-Sykes test, the most rigorous antiseptic test available, and it has proved effective, both in vitro and in vivo, against Candida albicans, Staphylococcus aureus, E. coli, ringworm, and streptococcus bacteria, and in vitro against *pseudomonas aeruginosa* (bluepus organism), pneumococcus, and diphtheria, among others.

Source: "Tea Tree Oil as an Effective Preservative," *Tea Tree Oil News*, Ballina, NSW, Australia, Issue 3, May 1995.

Most cosmetic products do not contain "all natural" ingredients; a preservative is added to keep bacteria and fungi from forming, which shorten the shelf life of the product. At a 1995 In-Cosmetics Conference in Paris, France, tea tree oil was demonstrated to be an effective preservative. A number of cosmetic formulations were examined using a pharmaceutical grade tea tree oil in 0.5% concentration. The strong scent of tea tree oil can be eliminated using this concentration. The British Pharmacopoeia 1993 Topical Protocol was used as the guideline for this study, and also included E. Coli which complied with the BP and the USP XX11 tests. This study shows that tea tree oil can be used in cosmetics as a safe alternative preservative, without any artificial ingredients.

Source: Blackwell, Rosalind. "An Insight into Aromatic Oils: Lavender and Tea Tree," *British Journal of Phytotherapy,* Vol. 2, No.1, 1991, ppg. 25-30.

Research reports indicate that tea tree oil can be particularly effective when taken internally against Candida albicans infection in the gut. For further information about this research, see: Pénoël, D., "The Place of Essential Oil of Melaleuca alternifolia in Aromatic Medicine." Paper presented at the Symposium on Tea Tree oil, Macer University, Sydney, Australia, 1990, or: Pénoël, D., Franchomme, P., *L'Aromatherapie Exactement.* Roger Jollois, Paris, 1990.

Toxicity Reports

Karen Cutter, a naturopath in Sydney, Australia, took 120 drops of tea tree oil daily for more than three months to demonstrate that her recommended dosages to patients associated with AIDS and systemic candida—60 drops daily over six months time—produced no side-effects. However, *this type of treatment is not recommended unless under a physician's care.*

Source: "Toxicity of the Essential Oil of Melaleuca alternifolia or Tea Tree Oil," *Clinical Toxicology,* 33a: (2), 193-194 (1995).

Tea tree oil contains as many as 100 organic compounds. The Australian standard (AS 2782-1985) only mentions two of those compounds: terpinen-4-ol, an antimicrobial component comprising 30% of the oil, and 1,8-cineole not to exceed 15%. The role of cineole is less clearly defined and has been known to be a skin irritant, especially at higher percentages. Also, there is little information available on the remaining compounds. There are a multitude of tea tree oil products in the marketplace now, and the problem is determining precise data on toxicity. Given the lipophilic nature of tea tree oil and its skin penetrating properties, toxicity is possible.

Source: *Tea Tree Oil News*. August/September/October 1996. Toxicology studies conducted on behalf of the Australian Tea Tree Oil Industry Association in the late 1980's indicated that neat (100%) tea tree oil has an oral LD_{50} in rats of 1700 mg / kg and may have some mild toxic effects if taken internally. It is therefore not recommended that neat tea tree oil be used for internal applications. Diluted, it can be used in mouthwashes, toothpastes, lozenges, lip balms, and for treatment of cold sores.

Source: Del Beccaro, Mark A., M.D., Department of Pediatrics, Children's Hospital & Medical Center, University of Washington, Seattle, WA 98105.[18]

A 17-month-old male ingested less than 10 ml. (approx. 1/3 oz.) of 100% pure Australian tea tree oil. Approximately 10 minutes after the ingestion, the child became sleepy, appeared unsteady, and was unable to sit or walk. There was no difficulty in breathing. The child was taken to an emergency clinic and was noted to be ataxic (lacking muscle control), and somewhat 'fussy.' He was admitted to the hospital for observation, and was free of symptoms within three hours. Other than a dose of activated charcoal, no treatment was given.

Source: Jacobs, M.R., C.S. Hornfeldt. *Journal of Toxicology - Clinical Toxicology*, 1994. 32(4):461-4. Comment by C.F. Carson, B.Sc.Hons and T.V. Riley, Ph.D. in: *Journal of Toxicology - Clinical Toxicology*, 1995. 33(2):193-4.

In one study, dermatitis caused by topical application of tea tree oil was exacerbated by ingestion. In another case, a 60-year-old man ingested half a teaspoon of tea tree oil, resulting in a "dramatic rash" and feeling "unwell," though the patient had taken tea tree oil on a number of prior occasions with no noticeable ill effects. In a third case, ingesting half a cup of tea tree oil resulted in a comatose state for 12 hours, followed by 36 hours in semi-conscious state.

---

[18]*Veterinary and Human Toxicology* 37 (6), December 1995.

Source: Jacobs, M.R., C.S. Hornfeldt. *Journal of Toxicology - Clinical Toxicology*, 1994. 32(4):461-4. Comment in: *Journal of Toxicology - Clinical Toxicology*, 1995. 33(2):193-4.

A 23-month-old child ingested less than 10 ml of T36-C7 (a commercial product containing 100% melaleuca oil). Within thirty minutes, the child was unable to walk. He was taken to a hospital and his condition improved; within 5 hours of ingestion he was free of symptoms. Melaleuca oil contains 50-60% terpenes and related alcohols. Clinical experience with products containing melaleuca oil is limited; however, this case report suggests that ingestion of a modest amount of a concentrated form of this oil may produce signs of toxicity.

Source: Knight, T.E., M.D., B.M. Hausen, Ph.D. "Melaleuca oil (tea tree oil) dermatitis." *Journal of the American Academy of Dermatology*, 1994. Mar. 30(3):423-7.

Over a three-year period, seven patients were patch-tested with Finn Chambers to a 1% solution (vol/vol) of Melaleuca oil and 1% solutions (vol/vol) of 11 constituent compounds. Purpose of the trial was to determine which constituent compounds of Melaleuca oil were responsible for allergic contact eczema in these patients. All patients had been applying a commercially-available 100% tea tree oil for skin conditions such as foot fungus, insect bites, rashes, dog scratches, and "pimples" of the legs. All patients initially had an eczematous dermatitis consisting of ill-defined plaques of erythema, edema, and scaling. Of the seven patients reactive to the 1% Melaleuca oil solution, six reacted to limonene, five to alpha-terpinene and aromadendrene, two to terpinen-4-ol, and one each to p-cymene and alpha-phellandrene. All patients had used the pure (100%) melaleuca oil on already damaged skin. Other melaleuca products containing lower concentrations of the oil and used on healthy skin may cause no sensitivity reactions.

Source: van der Valk, P.G., A.C. de Groot, D.P. Bruynzeel, P.J. Coenraads, J.W. Weijland. "Allergic contact eczema due to 'tea tree' oil." [Dutch] *Nederlands Tijdschrift voor Geneeskunde*, 1994. Apr. 16;138(16):823-5.

In four patients, three women aged 45, 29, and 52 years, and a man aged 45 years, allergic contact dermatitis due to 'tea tree' oil was diagnosed. The tea tree oil available in the Netherlands is distilled from the Melaleuca alternifolia and mainly contains eucalyptol. Eucalyptol is probably the most important allergen.

Source: "Toxicity of Melaleuca Oil and Related Essential Oils Applied topically on Dogs and Cats." *Veterinary and Human Toxicology*, 36(2) April 1994.

Cats and dogs: The most typical clinical signs of tea tree oil toxicity in animals include depression, muscle tremors, incoordination, and weakness. These symptoms have generally occurred with inappropriate or erroneous use of tea tree oil products; often with topical application of insecticidal dips 10-20 times the recommended concentrations. Thus, concentrations of tea tree oil beyond those recommended by the manufacturer can cause clinical signs of toxicosis in dogs and cats.

Source: Tisserand, Robert. *The International Journal of Aromatherapy*, February 1988. Referenced in article by Frank Murray, "Vitamins/ Supplements," *Better Nutrition for Today's Living*, Vol. 56, No. 4, April 1994.

The chemical content of tea tree oil has an unusually high content of terpinen-4-ol, an alcohol that constitutes some 35% of the best-quality oils. Tisserand states that there is no recorded toxicity data on tea tree oil, but the aforementioned alcohol gives the oil a toxicity of between 3 and 5—"a completely safe rating."

Safety Data

Identification

Product Name: Oil of Melaleuca alternifolia
Synonyms: Tea Tree Oil
Chemical Composition: Essential oil containing terpinen-4-ol, 1,8-cineole, p-cymene, etc.

Physical and Chemical Composition Data

Physical State: Liquid
Color: Colorless to pale yellow
Odor: Myristic
Specific Gravity: 20/20° C: 0.890 to 0.906
Refractive Index   At 20° C: 1.475 to 1.482
Solubility: Insoluble in water/soluble in alcohol
Boiling Point: Not determined
Vapor Density: (Air=1) >1
Saponification Value: 2-3
1,8 Cineole Content: Shall not exceed 10%
Terpinen-4-ol content: Shall be at least 36%

Fire and Explosion Hazard Data

Flash Point (open cup):   140° C
Extinguishing Media: Dry chemical foam
Special Fire Fighting
  Procedures: None known
Unusual Fire &
  Explosion Hazards: None known

Reactivity Data

Stability: Presents no significant reactivity hazard, stable even at elevated temperatures and pressures.

Incompatibility:	Solvent—avoid contact with plastics, oil based paints, ink, etc., or storage in plastic containers.
Hazardous Polymerization:	Does not occur.

Toxicity and Health Hazard Data

Toxicity:	No cases of acute or chronic toxicity reported. See Toxicity Reports, pages 70-73 for current data.
Health Hazards:	See Clinical Research data, pages 65-70.
First Aid:	Eye contact—irrigate with water. Skin irritation—wash with mild soap and water. Ingestion—drink copious quantities of water.

Personal Protection Information

Respiratory:	None required.
Ventilation:	Good room ventilation, local exhaust optional.
Protective Glove:	Oil resistant gloves optional.
Eye Protection:	Safety glasses optional.
Other Protective Equipment:	None required.

Special Storage and Handling Precaution

Store in stainless steel or amber-colored glass containers. Up to 20% tea tree oil may be stored in Polypropylene, PVC, PET and some laminates, although stainless steel or amber glass is recommended. Bottles should be well capped and kept in cool place.

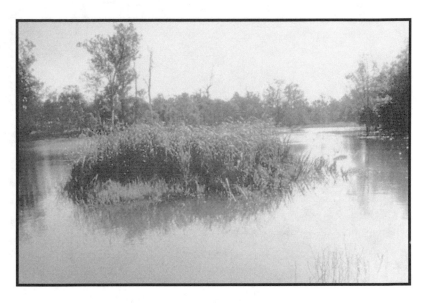

The Natural Habitat of Melaleuca alternifolia (Tea Trees)

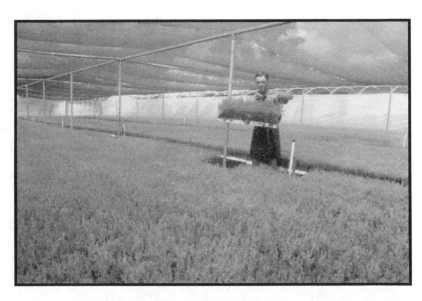

Nursery: Seedlings in Controlled Environment
Close to Planting Out Stage

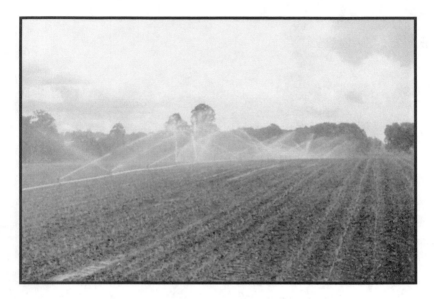

Irrigation of Cultivated Plants

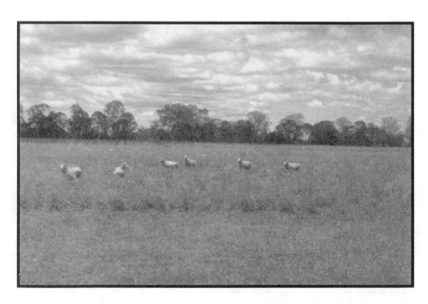

Sheep are Used to Control Weeds in Place of Chemicals

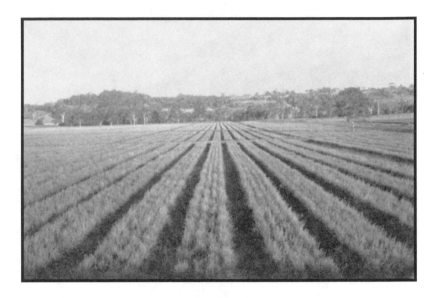

Plantation Scene - Trees Ready for Harvest

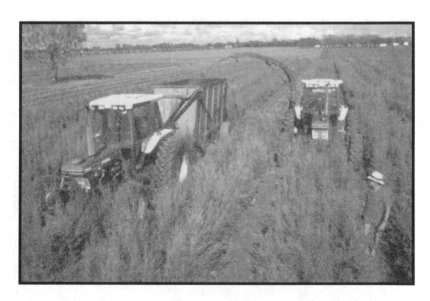

Harvesting Trees
Regrowth is Harvested Every 12 Months

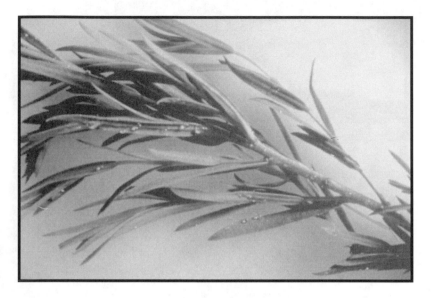

Tea Tree Leaves With Drops of Oil

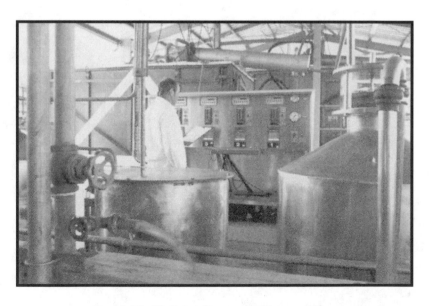

Steam Distillation of Leaves to Extract Oil

Appendix A

Glossary of Terms

Antiseptic-A solution used to clean human and animal skin to prevent blood infection (sepsis).

Arthritis-Inflammation of joints. Swelling, redness of the skin, and impaired motion. Two types: 1) osteo; chronic disease involving joints, especially weight-bearing joints; 2) rheumatoid; chronic disease characterized by inflammatory changes in joints that may result in crippling.

Boil (Furuncle)-A localized swelling and inflammation of the skin resulting from the infection of a sebaceous gland.

Candida albicans-A small oval budding yeast-like fungus that resides in vagina, alimentary tract. May result in *candidiasis* occurring in moist areas of the body, mouth, lungs, vagina, skin, nails or intestines. When occurring in the mouth, it is commonly called *thrush*.

Carbuncles-A collection of boils with multiple draining channels. Caused by *staphylococcus aureaus*. Usually terminates in extensive sloughing of the skin. Characterized by a painful node covered by tight red skin that later becomes thin and discharges pus. Commonly found on nape of neck, upper back, or buttocks.

Cold Sore (Herpes Simplex)-A viral infection causing inflammation of the skin, usually on mouth or lips, and characterized by collections of small blisters.

Corn (Clavus)-Area of hard, thickened skin on or between toes. May form an inverted pyramid pressing into deeper skin layers, causing pain.

Cradle Cap-Dermatitis of a newborn, usually appearing on scalp, face, and head. Thick, yellowish crusted lesions will develop on the scalp and scaling will appear behind ears.

Dandruff-Flaking scalp which may be caused by infection, poor diet and blood circulation, inadequate nerve stimulation, or a yeast (Pityrosporum ovale) which lives on the scalp, and/or a fungus (trichoplyton spp).

Dermatitis-An inflammation of the skin caused by an outside agent. The skin is red and itchy, and small blisters may develop. Causes may include soaps or detergents, sunlight, allergies, or hot weather. In about 70% of the cases, a family history exists.

Gingivitis-Inflammation of the gums, redness, swelling, and bleeding.

Hemorrhoids (Piles)-Enlarged varicose veins in the wall of the anus, often caused by chronic constipation or diarrhea, heavy lifting, or labor during childbirth.

Keratolytic-Causing the peeling of the horny layer of the epidermis.

Lipophilic-Fat loving.

Nasal Ulcer-An open sore or lesion of the mucous membrane accompanied by sloughing of inflamed tissue.

Miscible - Make water soluble by adding alcohol.

Perionychia - A fungal infection on fingernails and/or toenails, due primarily to harsh detergents or acrylic or silk nail applications.

Plantar Wart (Verruca Plantaris)-Wart occurring in skin on sole of foot, usually at base of toes. Caused by a virus. Because of pressure, these warts are painful.

Poison Ivy-Dermatitis resulting from irritation or sensitization of the skin by the resin of the poison ivy plant. Reaction to poison ivy contact may appear several hours or several days afterwards. Moderate itching or burning sensation followed by small blisters. Blisters will usually burst and be followed by oozing and crusting.

Poison Oak-A climbing vine, related to poison ivy.

Pruritus-Intense itching of the skin.

Psoriasis-A chronic skin disease with itchy, scaly red patches forming on elbows, forearms, knees, legs, scalp, and other part of the body. Affects 1-2% of the population.

Rash-An eruption on the skin characterized by redness and welts with very little elevation.

Scabies (sarcoptes scabiei)-Skin infection caused by the itch mite. Severe itching (especially at night), red papules, and secondary infection. Female mite tunnels into the skin to lay eggs. Newly hatched eggs are passed from person to person. Common areas affected are the groin, penis, nipples, and skin between fingers. Clothing and bedding should be disinfected.

Shingles (Herpes Zoster)-Viral infection of the nervous system characterized by pain and blisters. Blistering usually subsides within a three-week period. The virus also causes chicken pox in children.

Sinusitis-Inflammation of one or more of the mucus-lined air spaces. It is often caused by infection spreading from the nose. Symptoms may include headache and tenderness.

Tick-A blood-sucking parasite belonging to the order of arthropods that includes mites. Tick bites can cause skin lesions.

Tropical Ulcer (Naga Sore)-An indolent (inactive, painless) ulcer of lower extremities (feet or legs) usually occurring in hot, humid climates. May be due to bacteria, nutrition, or environment. A large, open sloughing sore usually develops.

Warts (Verruca)-A small (often hard) benign growth caused by a virus. Occurring on hands, fingers, face, elbows, and knees.

Appendix B

Tea Tree Information
and Specifications

Tea Tree Oil – Melaleuca alternifolia

Melaleuca alternifolia: common name "tea tree." A member of the laurel tree family, unusual variety indigenous to the east coast of New South Wales, Australia. Natural stands of trees usually found in low lying, swampy areas. Trees produced from seed are now being grown on plantations in the region. Seeds are quite small, and the quality of the seed affects the output of the plantation. Seedlings take seven to ten days to germinate in the summer months; when ten to fifteen cm. tall, they are transplanted.

The basis of any good tea tree oil crop is the genetic characteristics of the plant stock from which the oil is distilled. When the genetic blueprint for the highest quality essential oil is rigorously selected, there is no need to isolate or blend particular portions of the crop to produce an acceptable quality oil.

The only commercially viable method of extracting Australian tea tree oil is by distillation; most producers use steam distillation. Mechanical harvesters mulch the entire tree into large field bins which are then towed back to the distillery where, with the attachment of a steam hose to their base and a condenser mounted on their top, they become the distillation "pot." The oil contained in the leaves and terminal branchlets of the plant is readily vaporized by the steam. Upon cooling, the pure oil is separated from the condensate and without further processing is ready for analysis and shipment.

When a sufficient batch of oil is accumulated, retention and analysis samples are drawn off and sent to an independent accredited laboratory for gas chromatographic analysis. The laboratory also examines the physical constants of the oil (relative density, optical rotation, refractive index, and solubility). These are combined with the GC results of the components stipulated under ISO 4730 to give a full certificate of compliance to the international standard "Oil of Melaleuca Terpinen-4-ol Type (Tea Tree Oil)."

On at least one of the larger plantations, crops are ecologically sustainable with a very low reliance on chemical control measures. The large flocks of sheep that graze the plantation do an excellent job of grass and weed control, and at the same time convert unwanted plant matter to a soil-enhancing natural manure. Non-toxic vegetable extracts deter insects from feeding on the lush tea tree leaf, while careful husbandry prevents the plants being exposed to principal pests at the time they are most susceptible.

Legitimate "certified organic" tea tree oil is uncommon; producers did not exceed 1,500 kilograms (1.65 tons) of certified organic oil in the last harvest season, and this was three times the production of any previous years.

Essential Oil: steam-distilled essence from the root, bark, flower, and/or leaf of plants. Many oils are used in healing, aromatherapy, and culinary uses.

Composition of Tea Tree Essential Oil: Naturally-occurring essential oil, colorless or pale yellow. If discolorations appear, it usually indicates an inferior distillation process. Impurities and weeds in the distillation process may also affect the color. The oil is distilled from leaves of Melaleuca alternifolia, consisting chiefly of terpinenes, cymenes, pinenes, terpineols, cineole, sesquiterpenes, and sequiterpene alcohols. Pleasant characteristic odor with a terebinthinate taste. If odor is strong and varies from batch to batch, it may indicate impurities at the time of distillation.

Action: Pure tea tree oil conforming to Australian standard A.S.D. 175, revised 1985 (AS 2782-1985) and 1996 (ISO 4730) is a powerful broad-range antiseptic, fungicide, and bactericide. The main component is terpinen-4-ol (T-4-ol). Optimal activity at 35-40% w/v. Its bacterial action is increased in the presence of blood, serum, pus, and necrotic tissue. It is able to penetrate deeply into infected tissue and pus, mix with these, and cause them to slough off while leaving a healthy surface. The oil has a very low toxicity, and is virtually a non-irritant even to sensitive tissues. Because of its lower cineole level, tea tree oil is less toxic and less irritating than eucalyptus oil. Be aware that some unknown eucalyptus oils have been blended with a synthetic form of terpinen-4-ol, which alters the chemical composition.

Indications: Cuts, scratches, abrasions, burns, sunburn, prickly heat, insect bites, scalds, allergic and itching dermatoses, napkin and cosmetic rashes, senile, anal and genital pruritus, and lesions caused by herpes simplex virus including herpes labialis and herpes progenitalis. Impetigo contagiosa, furunculosis, psoriasis, and infected seborrhoeic dermatitis. Ringworm of scalp (microsporum canis), tropical ringworm (triphyton), becubitis and stasis ulcers, paronychia, oral thrush (candidiasis), tinea pedis, bromidrosis, and infestation with head, body, or pubic lice. As a gargle, throat spray, and nasal spray. Treatment of cutaneous staphylococcal reservoirs, boils and pimples. Pyorrhea, gingivitis, halitosis, and bronchial and sinus congestion. Gynecological conditions such as trichonomal vaginitis, moniliasis, and endocervicitis.

Precautions: Pure oil will dissolve certain plastics. Store only in glass (preferably amber) containers in a cool place. Bulk tea tree oil holds up much better from damage, deterioration, and oxidization if initially stored and shipped in steel drums.

Extremely sensitive skin may need dilutions of the pure oil. Dilutions of 1:250 are still bacteriostatic against pathogenic streptococci and staphylococci, typhous, pneumococcus, and gonococcus.

See Chapter Three for additional precautions.

Weights and Measures/Conversion Table

(Australian common usage to U.S. common usage)

1 milliliter (ml)	=	0.0338/fl. ounce
10 milliliter	=	0.338/fl. ounce
1 kilogram (kg)	=	2.2046 pounds

Bibliography

Aromatic Thymes, Vol. 4, No. 2, 1996.

Australian Journal of Dentistry, August 1930.

Australian Journal of Pharmacy, Vol. 72, January 1991.

Balacs, Tony. *International Journal Of Aromatherapy,* Research Reports, P.O. Box 746, Hove, E. Sussex, BN3 3XA, England. Volume 7, No. 3, 1996.

Belaiche, P. "Germicidal Properties of the Essential Oil of Melaleuca alternifolia Related to Urinary Infections and Chronic Ideopathic Colibacillus." *Phytotherapy,* September 1985, No. 115, pp. 9-11.

Belaiche, P. "Treatment of Vaginal Infections of Candida albicans with the Essential Oil of Melaleuca alternifolia." *Phytotherapie,* Vol. 15, 1985.

Bishop, C.D. "Antiviral activity of the essential oil of Melaleuca alternifolia (Maiden and Betche) Cheel (Tea tree) against tobacco mosaic virus." *Journal of Essential Oil Research,* 1995, 7: 641-644.

Blackwell, Rosalind. "An Insight into Aromatic Oils: Lavender and Tea Tree" *British Journal of Phytotherapy,* Vol. 2, No.1, 1991, pp. 25-30.

Breeden, Stanley. "The First Australians" *National Geographic,* National Geographic Society, Washington, DC, February 1988.

Brown, Donald J., N.D. "Tea Tree Oil for Bacterial Vaginosis and Monilial Vulvovaginitis" Townsend Letter for Doctors *Phytotherapy Review and Commentary,* May 1991.

Brown, Donald J., N.D. "Topical Tea Tree Oil for Nail Fungus" *HerbalGram,* Austin, TX. No. 35.

Buck, D.S., D.M. Nidorf, J.G. Addino. "Comparison of two topical preparations for the treatment of onychomycosis: Melaleuca alternifolia (tea tree) oil and clotrimazole." *Journal of Family Practice,* 1994. Jun; 38(6): 601-5.

Carson C.F. et al. "Susceptibility of Propionibacterium acnes to the essential oil of Melaleuca alternifolia." Letter in *Applied Microbiology,* 1994. 19(1):24-25.

Carson, C.F., B.D. Cookson, H.D. Farrelly, and T.V. Riley. "Susceptibility of methicillin-resistant *Staphylococcus aureus* to the essential oil of Melaleuca alternifolia." *Journal of Antimicrobial Chemotherapy,* 1995. 35:421-424.

Carson, C.F. and T.V. Riley. "Antimicrobial activity of the major components of the essential oil of Melaleuca alternifolia." *Journal of Applied Bacteriology,* 1995b. 78(3): 264-269.

Carson, C. F., B.Sc.Hons. and T.V. Riley, Ph.D. "Toxicity of the Essential Oil of Melaleuca Alternifolia or Tea Tree Oil." *Clinical Toxicology,* 33a: (2), 193-194 (1995).
Department of Microbiology, University of Western Australia.

Del Beccaro, Mark A., M.D., Department of Pediatrics, Children's Hospital and Medical Center, University of Washington, Seattle, WA. "Melaleuca Oil Poisoning in a 17-Month-Old";
Veterinary and Human Toxicology (newsletter, reports); VCS-Kansas State University, Manhattan, KS, Vol. 37 (6) December 1995, p. 557

Feinblatt, H.M. *Journal of the National Medical Association,* 1960. 52(1):32-34

Goldsborough, Robert E., F.C.S. "Ti-Tree Oil" *The Manufacturing Chemist,* February 1939, Vol. 57, pp. 45-58.

The International Journal of Aromatherapy, Vol. 7, No. 3, 1996.

Jacobs, M.R., and C.S. Hornfeldt; Comment in: *Journal of Toxicology - Clinical Toxicology,* 1995. 33(2):193-4. *Journal of Toxicology - Clinical Toxicology,* 1994. 32(4):461-4.

Knight, T.E., M.D., and B.M. Hausen, Ph.D. "Melaleuca oil (tea tree oil) dermatitis" *Journal of the American Academy of Dermatology,* 1994. Mar; 30(3):423-7.

McCaleb, Rob, "Tea Tree Oil and Antibiotic-Resistant Bacteria" *HerbalGram,* Austin, TX. No. 36, Spring 1996.
Medical Journal of Australia, Vol. 153, No. 8, October 15, 1990.

Murray, Frank. "Vitamins/Supplements" *Better Nutrition for Today's Living,* Vol. 56, No. 4, April 1994.

Newman, Marie. *Australia's Own Tea Tree Oil,* Mid-Richmond Historical Society, Coraki, NSW, Australia, 1992.

Pena, E. F. "Melaleuca alternifolia Oil, Uses for Trichomonal Vaginitis and Other Vaginal Infections." *Obstetrics and Gynecology,* June 1962.

Penfold, A.R., and F.R. Morrison. "Some Notes on the Essential Oil of Melaleuca alternifolia." *Australian Journal of Pharmacy,* March 30, 1930. *British Medical Journal,* 1933.

Puotinen, C.J. *Nature's Antiseptics: Tea Tree Oil and Grapefruit Seed Extract.* New Canaan, CT.; Keats Publishing, Inc., 1997.

Smith, Martha D., Patricia L. Navilliat. "A new protocol for antimicrobial testing of oils." *Journal of Microbiological Methods;* 28 (1997) 21-24.

Tea Tree Oil News; The Main Camp Tea Tree Oil Group Newsletter; Ballina, Australia. Issue 3, May 1995.

Tea Tree Oil News. August/September/October 1996.

Tea Tree Oil News. "A collaborative study between the Australian Tea Tree Oil Research Institute (ATTORI) and the University of Western Sydney (UWS)." November/December 1996 - January 1997.

Tisserand, Robert. "Australian Tea Tree Oil" *Aromatherapy for Everyone,* April 28, 1988.

van der Valk, P.G., A.C. de Groot, D.P. Bruynzeel, P.J. Coenraads, J.W. Weijland. "Allergic contact eczema due to 'tea tree' oil." [Dutch] *Nederlands Tijdschrift voor Geneeskunde,* 1994. Apr. 16; 138(16): 823-5.

Veterinary and Human Toxicology, 36(2) April 1994. "Toxicity of Melaleuca Oil and Related Essential Oils Applied Topically on Dogs and Cats."

Villiers, Alan, "Captain Cook: The Man Who Mapped the Pacific" *National Geographic,* National Geographic Society, Washington, DC, September 1971.

Walker, M. "Clinical Investigation of Australian Melaleuca alterni-folia for a variety of common foot problems." *Current Podiatry,* April 1972.

Weil, Andrew, M.D. *Natural Health, Natural Medicine,* Boston, MA; Houghton Mifflin Co., 1990.

Williams, Dr. Lyall, and Vicki Home. "A comparative study of some essential oils for potential use in topical applications for the treatment of the yeast *Candida albicans.*" School of Chemistry, Macquarie University, Sydney, NSW, Australia.

Resource Guide

A Directory of
Tea Tree Oil Products and Services

North American Companies

USA

A Natural Path
P.O. Box 70
Lewis, CO 81327
970-882-8888
Animal homeopathic kits, books.

Body Shop
The Body Shop by Mail
106 Iron Mountain Road
Mine Hill, NJ 07803
800-426-3922
Tea tree oil body care products.

Carter Wallace, Inc.
P.O. Box 1012
Cranbury, NJ 08512
609-655-6055 fax: 609-655-6305

Derma-E
9400 Lurline Avenue, #C-1
Chatsworth, CA 91311
800-521-3342
Tea tree oil hair and skin care products: shampoo, conditioner, tea tree oil vitamin E, tea tree oil cream.

Desert Essence
Ron Gerard, General Manager/Vice President Sales
9510 Vassar Ave., Unit A
Chatsworth, CA 91311
800-645-5768 fax: 818-705-8525
Tea tree oil health and body care products. Other brand name: Tea Tree Solutions.

Essential Care USA, Inc.
Division of Essential Resources, Sydney, Australia
Max Tessler, MD, President
661 Palisade Ave.
Englewood Cliffs, NJ 07632
201-567-9004 fax: 201-567-8853
Melaleuca oil products. Bulk oil; also retail markets, health and beauty aids.

InterNatural
P.O. Box 489
Twin Lakes, WI 53181
800-643-4221
website: www.internatural.com
Tea tree oil, herbs and natural health products. Over 14,000 items in stock.

Jason Natural Products
Jeffrey Light, President
8468 Warner Drive
Culver City, CA 90232
310-838-7543 fax: 310-838-9274
email: jnp@jason-natural.com
Tea tree oil health and body care products.

John Paul Mitchell Systems
9701 Wilshire Blvd., Suite 1205
Beverly Hills, CA 90212
310-248-3888
Body Care Products.

Other address:
26455 Golden Valley Road
Saugus, CA 91350
805-298-0400

Kali Press
P.O. Box 2169
Pagosa Springs, CO 81147
970-264-5200
order line: 888-999-5254
email: mail@kalipress.com
website: www.kalipress.com
Wholesale and distributor inquiries welcome.
Tea tree oil, essiac and other health products.

Marco Industries
3431 W. Thunderbird, Suite 144
Phoenix, AZ 85023
800-726-1612
602-789-7048
email: marco-lesi@juno.com
Manufactures 100% tea tree oil as a preservative and antiseptic; antiseptic herbal ointment, soothing cream in colloidal silver base, suppositories, douche; Convita tea tree oil toothpaste (New Zealand).

Rye Pharmaceuticals Pty. Ltd.
Beard Plaza
6540 Washington Street
Yountville, CA 94599
707-944-8090 fax: 707-944-8092
email: ryemkt@msn.com
Produces burn products since 1983; major product BURNAID, a tea tree oil compound available in tube, pump dispensers and sterile one-use dressings (burn blankets).

Thursday Plantation, Inc.
Michael Dean, President
330 Carillo St.
Santa Barbara, CA 93101
805-566-0354 fax: 805-566-9798
Tea tree products.

Trivent Chemical Company
4266 US Rt. One
Monmouth Junction, NJ 08852
Suppliers of raw material to cosmetic/pharmaceutical companies.

Water Jel Technologies
243 Veterans Blvd.
Carlstadt, NJ 07072
Peter D. Cohen, President
201-507-8300 fax: 201-507-8325
Medical supplies, tea tree burn blankets.

Herbs

American Botanical Council
P.O. Box 201660
Austin, TX 78720
512-331-8868 fax: 512-331-1924
email: custserv@herbalgram.org
website: www.herbalgram.org
Publishes *HerbalGram,* a quarterly journal geared toward health professionals, industry, and those interested in herb research, market conditions, and regulation. Also provides an Herbal Education Catalog, listing over 300 publications.

Aroma Vera
5901 Rodeo Rd.
Los Angeles, CA 90016-4312
800-669-9514 fax: 310-280-0395

Aura Cacia
101 Paymaster Rd.
Weaverville, CA 96093
800-437-3301 fax: 800-717-4372

Herb Pharm
20260 Williams Highway
Williams, OR 97544
800-348-4372 fax: 541-846-6112

Herb Research Foundation
1007 Pearl Street, Ste. 200
Boulder, CO 80302
303-449-2265 fax: 303-449-7849
Botanical research services. Co-publishes *HerbalGram.*

Lotus Light
P.O. Box 1008
Silver Lake, WI 53170
800-548-3824
Herbs, essential oils, natural products to wholesale customers only.

Starwest Botanicals, Inc.
11253 Trade Center Dr.
Rancho Cordova, CA 95742
916-638-8100
800-800-4372 fax: 916-638-8293
Tea tree oil to wholesale customers only.

Multi-Level Companies

Melaleuca Inc.
3910 S. Yellowstone Hwy.
Idaho Falls, ID 83402
208-522-0700 fax: 208-528-2090

Espial USA Ltd.
7045 South Fulton Street, Ste. 200
Englewood, CO 80112
800-695-5555 fax: 303-792-3933
Personal care products containing tea tree oil.

Canada

Australian Bodycare of Canada, Ltd.
Vancouver, BC
Canada
604-922-2562 fax: 604-922-2576
email: abc ca@istar.ca
website: www.beautynet.com/abc
Direct importer of tea tree oil, manufacturer and distrubutor of the
Professional Therapeutic Tea Tree Oil range of products.

Brueckner Group
Ron Jean
4717 14th Avenue
Markham, Ontario, L3S 3k3
Canada
905-479-2121 fax: 905-479-2122
Manufactures tea tree oil skin care products.

Australian Companies

The Australian Essential Oil Company Pty. Ltd.
W.R. (Bill) McGilvray, President
Brett J. Anderson, General Manager
575 Myall Creek Road
P.O. Box 158
Coraki, NSW 2471, Australia
tel: 61 266 832 124 fax: 61 266 832 603
email: wrmcg@ozemail.com.au   website: www.australessence.com
Bulk tea tree oil available in Organic "A," Eco-Harvest, or plantation-grown; premium, standard, or technical catetories. Currently ships 100 tons of essential oils to USA, Europe, and other parts of the world.

Bodycare Corp. Pty. Ltd.
Unit 4, 9-11 Villiers Drive
Currumbin, QLD, 4223, Australia
tel: 61 755 345 211 fax: 61 755 345 211
website: www.bodycare.com.au

Bronson & Jacobs Pty. Ltd.
William McCartney, Managing Director
Parkview Drive, Australia Centre
Homebush Bay NSW 2140, Australia
tel: 61 2 9394 3288 fax: 61 2 9394 3222
Plantation of 1700 acres, producing 50,000 kilos per annum. A major shareholder in Australian Plantations. Produces bulk oil. Exports to Europe and U.S.A., 60% into Europe.

Creatiqe Australia Pty. Ltd.
Rick Gruin, Managing Director
Christoph Nagel
PO Box 2420
Fortitude Valley BC
Queensland 4006, Australia
tel: 61 7 3254 1851 fax: 61 7 3254 1841
email: creatique@gil.com.au
Full range of natural personal care products.

Eureka Oils Pty. Ltd.
P.O. Box 85
Byron Bay, NSW 2481, Australia
tel: 61 2 6685 6333 fax: 61 2 6685 6313
Exports in a small way; does not have a plantation. Company carries 20% water miscible tea tree oil in 50 ml. size.

Gateway Pharmaceuticals
Mr. D. Bokeyar
274 Pennant Hills Road
P.O. Box 217
Thornleigh, NSW 2120, Australia
tel: 612 94 84 4764 fax: 612 98 75 3731
email: info@gatewaypharm.com.au
Bulk tea tree oil; veterinary and animal disinfectant products. Twenty hectares (49.4 acres); exports 5-6 tons of oil, mainly to Europe.

G.R. Davis Pty. Ltd.
Suite 3, 9 Apollo Street
Warriewood, NSW 2102, Australia
tel: 612 9 979 9844 fax: 612 99 79 9608
Exports bulk tea tree oil to U.S. and other countries; 30-50 tons per year. Plantation consists of 200 hectares (app. 494 acres). Produces bush oils from natural stands and markets oil for other growers.

Jurlique International Pty. Ltd.
Dr. Jurgen Klein, Director
Oborn Road
P.O. Box 522
Mt. Barker, South Australia, 5251
tel: 61 8 8391 0577
email: drklein@jurlique.com.au
website: www.jurlique.com.au
Skin care products.

Macquarie Plantations Pty. Ltd.
Leuk Andersen
17/7 Chapel Lane
Baulkiiam Hills, NSW 2153, Australia
tel: 61 2 9686 7891 fax: 61 2 9639 7831
Co-operative operations for smaller farms in the area (200 acres/ 3,000 trees). Research and development. Bulk oil shipped to U.S. - 12 tons; UK - 4 tons; Europe - 1 ton; SE Asia, India - 1 ton.

Main Camp Tea Tree Oil Group
(Level 1)
85 Tamar St.
P.O. Box 407
Ballina, NSW 2478, Australia
tel: 61 2 6686 3099 fax: 61 2 6686 2722
email: enquiry@maincamp.com.au
website: www.maincamp.com.au
Largest plantation in Australia. Produces 100 tons of oil from 50 million organically grown trees. Supplies three grades of tea tree oil: ISO standard grade; watersoluble; pharmaceutical grade.

Sunspirit Oils Pty. Ltd.
David Dane
6 Ti-tree Place
P.O. Box 85
Byron Bay NSW 2481, Australia
tel: 61 2 66 85 6 333 fax: 61 2 66 85 6 313
email: sunspirit@sunspirit.com.au
website: www.sunspirit.com.au
Exports 100% tea tree oil pure in 25 ml bottles and tea tree ointment in 50 gm (approx. 1.6 oz) in small numbers. They do not have a plantation.

Bulk Tea Tree Oil

Australian Holdings Inc.
William Branson
5855 Green Valley Circle #216
Culver City, CA 90230
310-348-1993 fax: 310-348-9074
800-763-7284

Essential Care USA, Div. of Essential Resources, Sydney, Australia (see USA Companies)

Mitech Laboratories Inc.
(& American Tea Tree Association)
Martha Smith
102 Haverford Rd
Pittsburgh, PA 15238-1620
412-967-9674 fax: 412-963-7747

International Sourcing Inc.
121 Pleasant Ave
Upper Saddle River, NJ 07458
201-934-8900

Lotus Brands, Inc.
P.O. Box 325
Twin Lakes, WI 53181
800-824-6396
email: lotusbrands@lotuspress.com
website: www.lotusbrands.com

Tea Tree Organizations

American Tea Tree Association (ATTA)
See Mitech

Australian Tea Tree Export and Marketing Ltd. (AUSTREAM)
Pat Bolster
P.O. Box 20
Tweed Heads, NSW 2485, Australia
tel: 61 2 6674 2925 fax: 61 2 6674 2475
email: attialtd@ozemail.com.au
A marketing and export company set up by the main industry producers in Australia, to market Australian tea tree oil internationally.

Australian Tea Tree Industry Association (ATTIA)
see address for AUSTREAM, above.

Australian Tea Tree Oil Research Institute (ATTORI)
Southern Cross University
Military Road
Lismore, NSW 2480, Australia
tel: 61 2 66 22 3211   fax: 61 2 66 22 3459
Recently, AUD $60 million was raised to build a new facility for research into the action and application of tea tree oil. The company responsible for this research facility is Main Camp Tea Tree Oil Group, located in New South Wales, Australia. The research will be carried out at Southern Cross University in Lismore, Australia with a staff of leading chemists and microbiologists; the advisory board will consist of authoritative people in the fields of dermatology, pharmacology, chemistry, and genetics.

The Institute will establish clinical studies to validate claims from "in-vitro" studies and anecdotal information. Pharmaceutical and cosmetic products will be formulated incorporating Main Camp's pharmaceutical grade tea tree oil. These products will be licensed and made available to companies using their own brand name. Other research will include Main Camp pharmaceutical grade as an antimicrobial. This research may assist in tea tree oil becoming a mainstream therapeutic component.

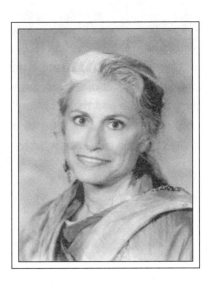

About the Author

*C*ynthia Olsen is the author of several books, a successful publisher, researcher, and speaker on complementary health, healing, ecology and spiritual awareness. In addition to her role as mother and grand-mother, she is a successful entrepreneur and business person and a lifelong supporter and exponent of holistic living. Her managerial experience in the health food industry in the 1980s led her to form an import company, becoming a leading figure in the introduction of Australian tea tree oil to the American health scene.

In 1990, Ms. Olsen founded Kali Press, a publishing house committed to works addressing the full spectrum of life awareness, with concentration on natural healing modalities. Her book *"Essiac: A Native Herbal Cancer Remedy,"* won the Small Press Book Award in 1997. As a result of her research into this remarkable herbal treatment,

Ms. Olsen and Kali Press participated in a program to bring its benefits to the Second Mesa Pueblo of the Hopi Nation.

Ms. Olsen's books have been translated into a number of languages. She has appeared on television, radio, and has addressed various conventions and meetings on health and natural living.

From her Colorado home, she continues to actively pursue her varied interests in nature and the spirit of joyful living.

Index

A

A Natural Path, 33
aborigines, x, 1
abrasions, 20
abscesses
  in cats and dogs, 36
aches, 23, 40
acne, x, 17, 47, 53, 62, 66
  study, 60, 66
action of tea tree oil, 83
after shave, 20
AIDS, 42, 43, 70
air conditioning systems, x, 68
allergies, 42
  in animals, from fleas, 32, 54
animal studies, 64
  hair loss, 64

meoestral vs. tea tree oil, 65
prednisolone vs. tea tree oil,
  65
toxicity, 73
animals
  abscesses, puncture wounds,
    35, 36
  dental hygiene
    excessive salivation, 37
    gum disease, 37
  fleas, 35, 54
  foul breath, 37
  horses, 37
  hot spots, 35, 54
  joint and muscle disorders, 36
  lice, 34

animals (continued)
   mange, 34
   parasites
      repellent for, 35, 36
   ringworm
      disinfection, 34
      treatment, 34
   skin conditions, 33, 54
      dermatitis, 33
      rashes, 33
      sunburn, 33
      vaccination sites, 33
      warts, 33
   sore muscles, 36
   tea tree oil insect repellent, 35
antifungal, 47, 59, 68
antimicrobial, 66, 67, 70
antimicrobial activity of tea tree
   oil, study of, 66
antiseptic, x, 47, 53, 77, 83
antiseptic cream, 53
aroma, 5
aromatherapy, 52, 82
arthritis, 23, 43, 77
   in animals, 36
athlete's foot, 47, 48, 58
ATTA
   American Tea Tree Associa-
      tion, 11, 100
ATTIA
   Australian Tea Tree Industry
      Association, 10, 100
ATTORI, 101
AUSTREAM, 100
Australia, ix–xi
Australian standard, 6, 10,
   11, 70. See also ISO
   International Standard

B

baby care, 23
   breast feeding, 23
   colds, 23
   cradle cap, 24
   diaper cleanser/deodorant, 24
   diaper rash, 24, 26
   disinfectant, 24
   ear infections, 24
   insect bites, 24
   skin rashes, 24, 26
bacteria, 4, 47, 50, 51, 59, 65,
   68, 69, 80
   tea tree oil active against, x
bacterial vaginosis, 62
bactericide, 83
bad breath, 40
baldness, 22
Banks, Joseph, 1
bath: tea tree oil in, 13, 23, 25,
   48, 52
Belaiche, Paul, 59
benzoyl peroxide
   study of tea tree oil vs., 60
biodegradable
   cleaning products, 55
bites
   animal, 20
   insect, 18
black walnut
   use with tea tree oil, 32
bleeding gums, 51, 54
blended oil, 10
boils, 77
   study of tea tree oil against, 58
   treatment for, 17
breast feeding, 23
bronchitis, 16

bruises, 23, 40
bulk oil, 10
burns, treatment for, 17
    burn salve, 17
bush oil, 6
bush still, 8

C

cajuput, 11
    use of oil with tea tree oil, 32
candida, 3, 53, 57
    systemic, 70
Candida albicans, 77
    study of tea tree oil against,
        59, 68
canker sores, 14, 62
carbolic acid, 2, 52
carbuncles, 78
cats
    fleas, 32
    ringworm, 32, 33
    skin conditions, 32, 33
cavities, 51
certificate of analysis, 11
cervicitis, 58
chemical composition, 74
chest conditions
    bronchial congestion, 16
    emphysema, 16
chicken pox, 41
chiropractors, 55
cineole, 6, 83
cloning, 4
clotrimazole, 63
cold sores, 14, 42, 48, 71, 78
cold-pressed oil, 13
colds, 40
    coughs, 16

head cold, 16
    in babies, 23
composition of tea tree oil, 83
compounds, 6
compresses, 52
contact dermatitis, 73
Cook, Captain James, 1
corns and callouses, 48, 58, 78
cosmetics, 47, 69
coughs, 16
cradle cap, 24, 50, 78
creams and lotions, 52, 53
cuts, 20, 40
    from coral, 19
    from shaving, 20
cutters, 7
cymene, 3, 83
cystitis, 59
    study of, 59

D

damaged skin, 47
dandruff, 22, 50, 78
debridement, 63
dehydration of the skin, 44
dental hygiene, 51
    gum bleeding, 15
    mouthwash, 15
    toothpaste, 15
dental problems. See also
        gingivitis
    in dogs and cats, 37
dental surgery, 54
deodorant, 54
deodorizer, 24
dermatitis, 17, 48, 72, 78
deterioration, 84

diabetes, 62
  gangrene as outgrowth of, 3
diaper rash, 24
diffuser, 24, 52
dilution, 84
diphtheria, 69
distillation, 8, 82
dogs
  fleas, 32, 35
  skin conditions, 32, 33
douche, 25, 26, 53, 58
dry hair, 22
dry skin, 48

E

E. coli, 67, 69
ears
  earaches, 14
  earaches in children, 24
eczema, 17, 62, 73
emphysema, 16
Escherichia coli, 67
essential oils, 82, 83
  mixing with other oils, alcohol,
    52
eucalyptus, 5
  oil of, 83
eyes
  styes, 15

F

face and body care, 48
facial masks, 52
FDA, 11
  recognition of tea tree oil, 67
fire and explosion hazard, 74
fleas, 32, 35
  prevention of, 32

tea tree oil in pet shampoos, 35
  skin conditions from, 35
foot conditions, 13, 58
  athlete's foot, 21
  callouses, 21
  corns, 21
  odor, 21
  study of tea tree oil in, 58
formulas, 58
foul breath, 37
fungicide, x, 52, 83

G

gangrene, 3
gas chromatographic analysis, 82
geriatric test, 62
  diabetic patients, 62
  skin conditions, 62
germicidal soap, 55
gingivitis, 3, 15, 54, 78
gynecological conditions, 3

H

hair and scalp, 22
  dandruff, 22
  dry hair, 22
  head lice, 22
  itchy scalp, 22, 41
  oily hair, 22
  thinning hair, 22
hair care, 50
hair thinning and loss, 50
hair treatments for children, 50
halitosis, 40, 54
harvesting, 7
head lice, 22, 51
hemorrhoids, 25, 53, 78

herpes lesions, 25
herpes simplex blisters, 41, 62
history, 1. *See also* World War II
hives, 18
horses, tea tree oil for, 37
humidifier
    tea tree oil in, 13

I

indications, 83
industrial grade, x
infections
    pus-filled, 3
ingestion, 26, 71
insect bites, 44
    in babies, 24
insect repellent, 36
ISO International Standard, 11
    See also Australian standard
    certificate of analysis, 12
    specifications for, 11

K

Kanuka, 11
kilogram, 83

L

Legionella pneumophila, 68
Legionnaire's Disease, 55, 68
lice
    preventing spread of, 22
    treatment for, 22
liniment, 36
lozenges, 71
lungs
    emphysema, 16

M

Main Camp Tea Tree Oil Group,
    9, 68
mange, 34
Manuka, 11
massage
    tea tree oil with, 52
Melaleuca alternifolia, 10, 81
Melasol, 59
methods of use. *See* humidifier:
    bath: creams and lotions
    pure oil, 14
    with cold-pressed oil, 13
metronidazole, 60
milliliter, 83
miscible, 57, 79
mold, x
monilia
    of throat, mouth, 62
    rashes of skin, 62
mosquito bites, 42
mouth conditions, 3
    bad breath, 15
    canker sores, 14
    chapped lips, 14
    cold sores, 14
    gingivitis, 15
    mouth ulcers, 14
    plaque, 15
    sore gums, 15, 51
    toothache, 15
mouthwash, 54, 71
multi-level companies
    tea tree oil products, 10
muscle aches, 23

N

nail fungus, 47, 49
  study of, 63
  topical preparations for
    tea tree oil vs. clotrimazole,
    63
nails
  infected nail bed, 3, 21
  stains, 49
nasal
  blocked, 14
  ulcers, 15, 79
naturopaths, 55
Nicotinia glutinosa, 68

O

onychomycosis, 63
oral hygiene, 3
organic tea tree oil, 82
ovarian cysts, 25
oxidation, 84

P

patch test, 27
Pena Study, 57. *See also* yeast
  infections
Penfold Study
  tea tree oil as antiseptic, 2
periodontal disease
  in animals, 37
  in humans, 15
perionychia, 3, 21, 79
personal care
  bikini waxing, 25
  hemorrhoids, 25
  herpes lesions, 25
  ovarian cysts, 25

vaginal cleansing, 25
vaginal infection, 26
pessary, 53, 60
pet shampoo, 54
pharmaceutical grade, x–xi
physical composition of tea tree
  oil, 74
pinenes, 3, 83
Pityrosporum ovale, 50
plantar warts, 19, 21, 79
plantations, 8
plaque, 15, 43, 51, 54
plastics, storing oil in, 84
pneumococcus, 69
poison ivy, 79
  treatment of, 18
poison oak
  treatment of, 18, 79
precautions, 26, 84
  alcohol and essential oils, 27
  babies' skin, 26
  children, 26
  eyes, 26
  ingestion, 26
  patch test, 26
  pregnancy, 27
  sensitive areas, skin, 26
preservative
  tea tree oil as, 69
production, 9
  hectare, 9
  seedlings, producing trees
    from, 9
  tonnage, 9
properties, xi
Protex, 55
pruritus, 61, 79
Pseudomonas aeruginosa, 67, 69

psoriasis, 18, 79
puncture wounds
  in animals, 35
pus, 58
pustules
  infected, 62
pyorrhea, 3, 54

R

rash, 18, 24, 79
razor burns, 54
receding gums, 43
ringworm, 19
  cajuput and black walnut oil in
    treatment of, 32
  in animals, 32, 34

S

safety data, 74
  chemical composition, 74
  fire and explosion hazard, 74
  health hazards, 75
  incompatibility, 75
  personal protection
    protective eyewear, 75
    protective glove, 75
    respiratory, 75
    ventilation, 75
  physical composition, 74
  reactivity data, 74
  storage and handling, 75
sarcoid, 44
scabies, 79
scalp, 41
  itchy scalp, 22
seedlings
  growing trees from, 9, 81

sensitive skin, 41
sesquiterpene [alcohol], 83
shampoo, 53
shaving, 48
shelf life, 27
shingles, 19, 79
sinus
  blocked, 14
sinusitis, 80
skin conditions, 33
  acne, 17
  boils, 17
  burns, 17
  coral cuts, 19
  dermatitis, 17
  eczema, 17
  hives, 17
  leeches, ticks, 18
  leg ulcers, 18
  plantar warts, 19
  poison ivy, 18
  psoriasis, 18
  rashes, 18
  ringworm, 18
  sore nipples, 19
  stings/bites, 18, 19
  study of tea tree oil against, 61
  sunburn, 19
skin eruptions, 40
soaps, 53
solvent, tea tree oil as, 75
sore muscles
  in dogs and cats, 36
sore nipples
  treatment of, 19
sore throat, 43
sprains, 23
standard grade, x–xi

Staphylococcus aureus, 65, 67
  study of tea tree oil against, 65
stings, 19
storage, 27, 53, 75
sun screens, 55
sunburn, 19, 41
synthetic drugs, 4

T

tampons, 26, 44
tea tree oil
  as a renewable resource, xi
  information and specifications, 81
  internal use of, 70
  products containing, 55
  testing of, 67
tea trees, 6
  growing, 9
terpenes, 3
terpinen-4-ol, 6
terpinene, 3, 83
terpineol, 3, 83
throat, sore, 3, 16
thrush, 16
Ti-Tree, 11
ticks, 18, 35, 80
tinea, 3
  barbae, 62
  cruris, 62
  pedis, 62
Tisserand, Robert
  aromatherapy, 52
tobacco mosaic virus
  study of tea tree oil against, 68
toothache, 15
toothpaste, 54, 71

toxicity, 48, 70, 71, 75
  allergic reaction in skin application, 72, 73
  and alcohol content, 73
  in animals, 73
  ingestion by 17-month-old, 71
  ingestion by 23-month-old, 72
  tea tree oil applied topically on dogs and cats, 73
trichomonal vaginitis, 57
trichoplyton spp, 50
tropical ulcer, 19, 80
typhoid bacilli, 3

V

vaginal cleansing, 25, 40
vaginal conditions, 26, 69
vaporizer, 13
  tea tree oil in, 24, 52
viridflorene, 5

W

warts, 19, 43, 80
  in animals, 33
waxing, 48
weed control, 82
weights and measures, 84
whiteheads, 40
World War II, 4
wounds, 20, 35
  cleansing, 40
  dressing, 3

Y

yeast, 50, 77
yeast infections, 53, 57

Other Titles from Lotus Press

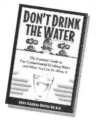

Don't Drink the Water:
The Essentail Guide to Our Contaminated Drinking Water and What You Can Do About It

Lono Kahuna Kupua Ho'ala

Additional copies of *Don't Drink the Water* are available through Lotus Press.

Trade Paper ISBN 0-962888-29-X 112 pp $11.95

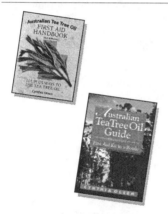

The Authoritative Tea Tree Oil Reference Books

Cynthia Olsen

Author/researcher Cynthia Olsen presents the most comprehensive books on this ancient remedy. The *Australian Tea Tree Oil First Aid Handbook* describes 101 ways to use tea tree oil (*Melaleuca alternifolia*) from head to toe—a must for users of this "first aid kit in a bottle." The new *Australian Tea Tree Oil Guide* contains updated information which includes production, quality control, research and a practitioners section.

Australian Tea Tree Oil First Aid Handbook, 2nd Edition
Trade Paper ISBN 1-890941-02-6 96 pp $6.95

Australian Tea Tree Oil Guide, 3rd Edition
Trade Paper ISBN 1-890941-01-8 140 pp $9.95

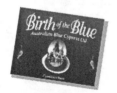

Birth of the Blue: Australian Blue Cypress Oil
Cynthia Olsen

A new, magnificent, aqua colored essential oil from the Northern Territory of Australia. Selected as the "Essence of the Sydney 2000 Summer Olympics." Blue Cypress Oil's woody fragrance has soothing and moisturizing skin benefits.

Trade Paper ISBN 1-890941-04-2 88 pp $7.95

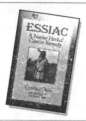

Essiac: A Native Herbal Cancer Remedy, 2nd Edition
Cynthia Olsen

The remarkable story of Canadian nurse Rene Caisse and her herbal anti-cancer formula.

Winner of the Small Press Book Award

Trade Paper ISBN 1-890941-00-X 144 pp $12.50

Available at bookstores and natural food stores nationwide or order your copy directly by sending the cost of the book(s) plus $2.50 shipping/handling ($.75 s/h for each additional copy ordered at the same time) to:

Lotus Press, PO Box 325, Dept. TTG, Twin Lakes, WI 53181 USA

toll free order line: 800 824 6396   office phone: 262 889 8561   office fax: 262 889 2461
email: lotuspress@lotuspress.com   web site: www.lotuspress.com

Lotus Press is the publisher of a wide range of books and software in the field of alternative health, including Ayurveda, Chinese medicine, herbology, aromatherapy, Reiki and energetic healing modalities. Request our free book catalog.

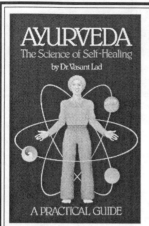
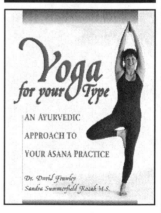

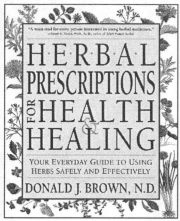
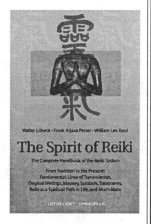

Neem
The Ultimate Herb
by John Conrick

Neem, The Ultimate Herb is the most comprehensive book about neem, the world's most amazing plant. This book provides easy-to-understand instructions for using neem along with credible scientific evidence as to its effectiveness. After finishing this book, you will understand and appreciate the amazing qualities found in neem. You will also be able to more intelligently select quality neem products for your own use.

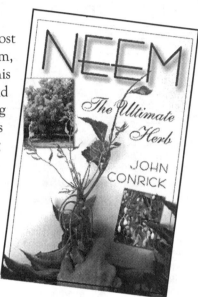

Trade Paper   ISBN 0-910261-32-6   184 pp   pb $12.95

Available at bookstores and natural food stores nationwide or order your copy directly by sending $12.95 plus $2.50 shipping/handling ($.75 s/h for each additional copy ordered at the same time) to:

Lotus Press, PO Box 325, Dept. TTG, Twin Lakes, WI 53181 USA
toll free order line: 800 824 6396   office phone: 262 889 8561
office fax: 262 889 2461   email: lotuspress@lotuspress.com
web site: www.lotuspress.com

Lotus Press is the publisher of a wide range of books and software in the field of alternative health, including Ayurveda, Chinese medicine, herbology, aromatherapy, Reiki and energetic healing modalities. Request our free book catalog.

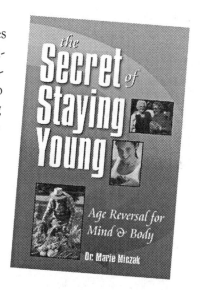

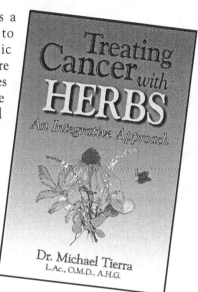